OCCLUSION AND CLINICAL PRACTICE

AN EVIDENCE-BASED APPROACH

Commissioning Editor: Michael Parkinson
Project Development Manager: Janice Urquhart
Project Manager: Nancy Arnott
Designer: Erik Bigland
Illustrator: Robert Britton

OCCLUSION AND CLINICAL PRACTICE
AN EVIDENCE-BASED APPROACH

Edited by

Iven Klineberg AM RFD BSc MDS PhD FRACDS FDSRCS(Ed) FDSRCS(Eng) FICD

Professor of Prosthodontics, Faculty of Dentistry, Westmead Centre for Oral Health, Westmead, New South Wales, Australia

Rob Jagger BDS MScD FDSRCS

Reader and Consultant in Restorative Dentistry, Department of Adult Dental Health, UWCM Dental School, Cardiff, Wales, UK

Foreword by

Professor Nairn Wilson BDS MSc PhD FDSRCS DRDRCS

Dean and Head of School, GKT Dental Institute, King's College, London, UK

wright

EDINBURGH LONDON NEW YORK OXFORD PHILADELPHIA ST LOUIS SYDNEY TORONTO
2004

WRIGHT
An imprint of Elsevier Limited

First published 2004

ISBN 0 7236 1092 4

British Library Cataloguing in Publication Data
A catalogue record for this book is available from the British Library

Library of Congress Cataloging in Publication Data
A catalog record for this book is available from the Library of Congress

Notice
Medical knowledge is constantly changing. Standard safety precautions must be followed, but as new research and clinical experience broaden our knowledge, changes in treatment and drug therapy may become necessary or appropriate. Readers are advised to check the most current product information provided by the manufacturer of each drug to be administered to verify the recommended dose, the method and duration of administration, and contraindications. It is the responsibility of the practitioner, relying on experience and knowledge of the patient, to determine dosages and the best treatment for each individual patient. Neither the Publisher nor the editors and contributors assume any liability for any injury and/or damage to persons or property arising from this publication.
The Publisher

ELSEVIER SCIENCE your source for books, journals and multimedia in the health sciences
www.elsevierhealth.com

The publisher's policy is to use **paper manufactured from sustainable forests**

Printed in China

Foreword

It is a great honour to be asked to prepare a foreword for an important textbook. The task is made all the more pleasant when the book is one that I have enjoyed reading, wish I had been able to write, and look forward to having available for subsequent reference.

Occlusion is fundamental to the clinical practice of dentistry, yet many students and practitioners may admit to being uncertain, if not confused about relevant terminology, approaches to management and appropriate clinical procedures. Setting out the best available evidence on occlusion in a systematic, easy to read, authorative style, with chapter synopses, key points and helpful references, *Occlusion and Clinical Practice: An Evidence-Based Approach* enables the reader to build, or restore a solid foundation of knowledge of occlusion, spanning the complexities of the masticatory system, its assessment and management. This is an elegant, carefully crafted textbook, which more than fulfils its stated aims and the readers' expectations – a most valuable addition to any dental library or treasured collection of selected texts.

What else is special about *Occlusion and Clinical Practice: An Evidence-Based Approach?* Amongst this book's many attributes, it is exceedingly well written and produced in meticulous detail by a truly international team. The style is contemporary and consistent throughout, the illustrations are uniformly of a high quality and, despite being a multi-author volume, the text lends itself to selected reading – a bonus for those deprived of time and opportunity to read and enjoy the book from beginning to end.

Can I recommend this book to students and established practitioners alike? Yes, most certainly. There is something for everyone, and for most a rich resource of new knowledge and understanding of occlusion, together with practical guidance on relevant state-of-the-art clinical procedures.

The editors – Iven Klineberg and Rob Jagger, together with the exceptionally well qualified cast of contributors, are to be congratulated on a job well done. An outstanding book which is a most welcome and timely addition to existing literature.

Nairn Wilson   London 2003

Acknowledgements

We wish to acknowledge the support of colleagues who contributed chapters. Each one with their specialised knowledge in their respective field has provided a comprehensive picture of the biological framework of occlusion for clinical practice.

We are indebted to our students, both undergraduate and graduate for continuing to stimulate our interest and challenge our knowledge. This text is dedicated to them.

Special appreciation is due for the administrative expertise, personal interest and attention to detail at all stages of this project to Personal Assistant Mrs Tracey Bowerman, and to Ms Pat Skinner for her meticulous editorial support. Without these commitments, this work would not have been possible.

Preface and introduction

This text book reviews, updates and expands on an earlier work by Klineberg (1991). During the last decade dentistry has moved further from its mechanical beginning than ever before and now emphasises – in all disciplines, the biological basis of dental practice. Educational programmes of necessity need to reflect these fundamental changes in philosophy which were comprehensively presented in Dental Education at the Crossroads – Challenges and Change (Field 1995). In addition, the recognition of evidence-based dentistry has been a further stimulus to review our core values in education and practice; as has been the case in medicine (Sackett et al 1996).

In recognition of these needs, the authors aim to provide the reader with the best available evidence on occlusion and its clinical applications. The authors recognise that this is an important requirement of educational programmes and are mindful of the need for applying knowledge of occlusion in clinical practice.

Dental occlusion has been described as the way in which teeth contact. This however represents only a limited view and a modern understanding of occlusion includes the relationships of the teeth, jaw muscles and temporomandibular joints in function and dysfunction. Occlusion is of importance to the provision of comprehensive patient care. It is of relevance to all disciplines in dentistry.

Occlusion is of particular relevance to restorative dentistry and prosthodontics, where tooth restoration requires recognition of the importance of occlusal form and tooth contact patterns at an appropriate occlusal vertical dimension, for optimising jaw function. The occlusion is a focal point for orthodontic treatment, has a significant bearing on tooth mobility, and is an important consideration in treatment planning for maxillofacial reconstruction. In all these fields, an understanding of the importance of the occlusion is paramount for enhancing jaw function, defining lower face height and aesthetic needs, as key issues in optimising oral health. In addition to facial appearance, orofacial integrity is a crucial element for psycho-social wellbeing.

The text is divided into three parts:

Part 1: Biological Considerations of the Occlusion – which provides an overview of the functional biology of the jaw muscle system. Tooth relationships are of special importance in restoration and maintenance of oral function, and with interarch relationships of teeth, form the basis of functional integrity and jaw movement control. Growth and development provides the framework for understanding the interdependence of form and function, and together with the anatomy and pathophysiology of the temporomandibular joints and an understanding of jaw movement, defines the biological basis of occlusion. Dental treatment involving the alteration or replacement of tooth crowns and contacting surfaces, impacts directly on this biological milieu. Recognition of this interaction of form and function confirms the singular importance of careful management of the occlusion in the quest for developing or maintaining optimal oral health.

Part 2: Assessment of the Occlusion – summarises a clinical approach for clinical occlusal analysis and for evaluation of study casts as an indispensable part of treatment planning.

Part 3: Clinical Practice and the Occlusion – provides practical guidelines for clinical management of the occlusion in relation to temporomandibular joint and jaw muscles, periodontal health, orthodontic treatment, fixed and removable prosthodontic treatment, implant restoration, and defines the role of occlusal splints and occlusal adjustment.

This book has been written for senior dental undergraduates and dentists with a particular interest in prosthodontics and restorative dentistry. Each chapter contains key references and additional recommended reading, to encourage the reader to pursue further their area of special clinical interest.

The text and individual chapters are designed to:

a) provide an understanding of the framework within which occlusion is required in clinical practice;

b) provide clinical research information and where possible, biological justification for the clinical application of occlusion.

The authors realise however, that the evidence based on systematic clinical research and long-term clinical studies is weak in many aspects of the role of the occlusion in biological function and harmony. There is also lack of convincing evidence for a possible link of the occlusion with functional disorders of the jaw muscle system.

Clinical studies have, in general, not adequately addressed the issues of the importance of the occlusion and its pivotal links with form, function and psychosocial wellbeing. It is recognised that there has, in general, been no uniformity in clinical study design to allow data comparison. Study design has not consistently addressed issues of patient numbers, long-term follow up, blinding of clinical treatment options, bias and critical assessment of outcome measures. Carefully designed clinical trials are needed to provide treatment guidelines based on biological research and long-term clinical outcome studies of treatment procedures.

In the absence of appropriate clinical trials and long-term studies on clinical outcomes, clinical practice continues to be primarily based on clinical experience which is often tempered with clinical convenience (operator bias).

Evidence-based practice is important for medicine and dentistry to optimise treatment outcomes as the cornerstone of best practice. Evidence-based practice is based on the combination of:

a) high quality scientific and careful long-term clinical trials, which provide research evidence to support clinical decision making;

b) clinical experience is an essential component to allow appropriate interpretation of each patient's needs;

c) the ability to ask the right questions in searching for the appropriate information;

d) interpreting that information for application to a particular clinical problem; and

e) satisfying each patient's expectations, rather than providing a predetermined treatment protocol.

In the past, clinical experience has directed the path of clinical treatment, and the developing acknowledgement of an evidence-based practice approach is a welcome advance for clinical dentistry; it has already been embraced in clinical medicine.

Iven Klineberg
Rob Jagger

References

Klineberg I 1991 Occlusion: Principles and assessment. Wright, Oxford

Field M J (ed) 1995 Dental education at the crossroads – challenges and change. National Academy Press, Institute of Medicine, Washington

Sackett D L, Rosenberg W M C, Gray J A M, Haynes R B, Richardson W S, 1996 Evidence based medicine: What it is and what it isn't: It's about integrating individual clinical expertise and the best external evidence. British Medical Journal 312: 71–72

Contributors

Anthony Au BDs MDSc FRACDS
Private Practitioner, Turramurra, New South Wales, Australia

Merete Bakke DDS PhD DrOdont
Associate Professor, Department of Oral Function and Physiology, School of Dentistry, Copenhagen, Denmark

Gunnar Carlsson LDS OdontDr/PhD DrOdonthc FDSRDS(Eng)
Editor-in-chief, International Journal of Prosthodontics; Professor Emeritus, Department of Prosthetic Dentistry, Faculty of Odontology, Göteborg University, Sweden

Ali Darendelilar BDS PhD DipOrtho
Discipline of Orthodontics, Faculty of Dentistry, University of Sydney, New South Wales, Australia

Annmarie De Boever DDS
Department of Fixed Prosthodontics and Periodontology, Dental School, Universiteit Gent, Belgium

Jan De Boever DDS DMD PhD
Professor, Department of Fixed Prosthodontics and Periodontology, Dental School, Universiteit Gent, Belgium

John Hobkirk PhD BDS FDSRCS(Ed) FDSRCSEng DrMedHC MIPEM
Professor of Prosthetic Dentistry, Eastman Dental Institute for Oral Health Care Sciences, University College, University of London, UK

Rob Jagger BDS MScD FDSRCS
Reader and Consultant in Restorative Dentistry, Department of Adult Dental Health, UWCM Dental School, Cardiff, Wales, UK

Om Kharbanda BDS MDS MNAMS FICD
Head, Orthodontics Department, Westmead Centre for Oral Health, Westmead, New South Wales, Australia

Iven Klineberg AM RFD BSc MDS PhD FRACDS FDSRCS(Eng) FICD
Professor of Prosthodontics, Faculty of Dentistry, Professorial Unit, Westmead Centre for Oral Health, Westmead, New South Wales, Australia

Jeremy Knox BDS MScD PhD FDSRCS(Ed) MOrthRCS(Ed) FDS(Orth)
Department of Orthodontics, UWCM Dental School, Cardiff, Wales, UK

Greg Murray BDS MDS PhD FRACDS
Associate Professor, Faculty of Dentistry, Professorial Unit, Westmead Centre for Oral Health, Westmead, New South Wales, Australia

Sandro Palla Prof Dr med dent
Professor, Klinik für Kaufunktionsstörungen und Totalprothetik Zentrum für Zahn-, Mund- und Kieferhelkunde, Universität Zürich, Switzerland

Terry Walton BDS MDSc MS(Mich)
Private Practitioner, Sydney, New South Wales, Australia

Tom Wilkinson BDS MSc MDS
Private Practitioner, Adelaide, South Australia, Australia

Contents

BIOLOGICAL CONSIDERATIONS OF THE OCCLUSION

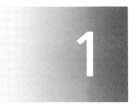

Interarch relationships of teeth

I. Klineberg

The term 'occlusion' represents a broader concept than the arrangements of teeth. Occlusion is the dynamic biological relationships of components of the masticatory system that control tooth contacts during function and dysfunction. It is essentially the integrated action of the jaw muscles, temporomandibular (TM) joints and teeth.

The essential characteristics of the system morphologically and physiologically are genetically determined (jaw muscle characteristics, jaw shape and size, tooth eruption sequence), and functional relationships mature during growth and development. However, once established, continual modification of the jaw muscle system occurs with function and parafunction.

Importantly, the influence of parafunction on tooth position and wear may be significant, with ongoing remodelling of bone and muscle allowing adaptation to prevailing circumstances, emphasising the dynamic nature of this complex biological system.

Synopsis

This chapter reviews relationships of teeth that are important in the clinical management of the occlusion. These include an understanding of tooth contact positions in the natural dentition and the clinical recordings of jaw position for treatment purposes. Occlusal relationships are summarised, recognising the prevailing divergent views in defining optimal jaw and tooth contact relationships. The implications of the variations that are described in population studies are considered, and their possible links with jaw muscle pain and temporomandibular disorders (TMDs) reviewed.

A summary statement on occlusal relationships emphasises the difficulty in defining optimum occlusal features. The border movement diagram is summarised as an important statement of historical development in the field, and as a useful conceptual tool for understanding border positions. Anterior and lateral guidance is defined in the light of research evidence, in conjunction with the emerging research evidence on mediotrusive contacts/ interferences. Features of the natural dentition are distinct from guidelines recommended for restoration of the occlusion.

There is a need for more carefully designed clinical studies, as much of what has been published does not present strong evidence for clarifying issues. It is encouraging, however, that more recently, systemic reviews (Clark et al 1999, Forssell et al 1999, Marklund & Wänmann 2000, Tsukiyama et al 2001) and controlled trials (Pullinger & Seligman 2000, Seligman & Pullinger 2000), some of which are randomised and blinded, have been reported. It is also recognised that human physiological studies of jaw and condyle position and movement, and electromyographic (EMG) studies, especially of deep jaw muscles, are technically demanding, and recruitment of subjects is often difficult. Notwithstanding these challenges, progress is being made in moving forward from our mechanical heritage to a recognition of the complexities of the biological system within which occlusal management is of clinical and psychosocial importance.

Key points

- Occlusion is the dynamic biological relationship of the components of the masticatory system that determine tooth relationships
- Intercuspal contact (IC) is the contact between the cusps, fossae and marginal ridges of opposing teeth
- Intercuspal position (ICP) is the position of the jaw when the teeth are in IC
- Maximum intercuspation (MI) is the contact of the teeth with maximum clenching
- Centric occlusion (CO) is the IC when the jaw and condyles are in centric relation
- ICP and CO are not usually the same tooth contact positions, that is, there is a slide from CO to ICP
- Median occlusal position (MOP) is a clinically determined tooth contact jaw position obtained by a 'snap' jaw closure from a jaw open position
- Retruded jaw position (RP) is the guided jaw position with the condyles in a physiologically acceptable position for recording transfer records
- Retruded contact position (RCP) is the tooth contact position when the jaw is in RP
- Centric relation (CR) is the guided jaw position where the condyles are located anterosuperiorly, in contact with the central bearing surface of the interarticular disc located against the articular eminence
- Postural jaw position (PJP) is the jaw position determined by the jaw muscles when the subject is standing or sitting upright, with variable space between the teeth
- Occlusal vertical dimension (OVD) is the vertical height of the lower third of the face with the teeth in ICP
- Lateral jaw positions:
  - Mediotrusive (non-working) side contact arises when the jaw is moved or guided to the opposite side, and the mediotrusive side moves medially, that is, towards the midline
  - Laterotrusive (working) side contact occurs when the jaw is moved or guided to the side, that is, laterally to the right or left. The tooth contacts on that side are termed laterotrusive (or working) contacts

- Bennett movement is a term that describes lateral movement of the condyle, that is, condyle movement to the laterotrusive (or working) side
- Bennett angle is the angle of the condyle formed with the sagittal plane on the mediotrusive side as the condyle moves forward downwards and medially
- Protrusive jaw movement describes a forward (straight line) jaw movement, and protrusive tooth contacts include incisal tooth contact

TOOTH CONTACTS AND JAW POSITIONS

The need to describe jaw and tooth positions accurately for treatment planning, writing of clinical reports and for laboratory prescriptions requires an understanding of the following customarily accepted descriptive terms:

- *Intercuspal contact (IC)* is the contact between the cusps, fossa and marginal ridges of opposing teeth.
- *Intercuspal position (ICP, IP)* is the position of the jaw when the teeth are in intercuspal contact (IC). Light IC occurs with light tooth contact; in this situation, the number and area of tooth contacts are less than with heavy tooth contact (clenching). ICP is the tooth contact position at the end of the closing phase and the beginning of the opening phase of mastication. Most natural occlusions indicate ICP contacts as a combination of flat and inclined surfaces or inclined planes with supporting cusp to opposing tooth fossa or marginal ridge. The greatest number of contacts occurs between molar teeth, and this decreases to 67% contacts on first bicuspids and 37% contacts on second bicuspids. Light to heavy biting approximately doubles the number of tooth contacts (Riise & Ericsson 1983).
- *Maximum intercuspation (MI)* occurs with clenching (heavy bite force), when the number and area of tooth contacts are greatest. The increase in number and area of tooth contacts occurs as a result of tooth compression within the periodontal space, which for individual teeth may be of the order of 100 μm in healthy periodontal tissues. With periodontal disease and periodontal bone loss, this may be greater.

The distinction between ICP and MI might appear to be of academic rather than clinical interest; however, the recognition of an increase in the number of tooth contacts is relevant when finalising anatomical tooth form for restorations, to ensure that with clenching the restoration is not too heavily loaded.

- *Centric occlusion (CO)* and ICP may be considered the same for clinical purposes; however, the *Glossary of Prosthodontic Terms* (Preston et al 1999) defines CO as the tooth contact position when the jaw is in centric relation. CO may or may not be the same tooth contact relationship as ICP. Tooth contacts (CO) when the jaw is in centric relation may be more retruded than at ICP. In an epidemiological study, Posselt (1952) determined that CO and ICP coincided in only approximately 10% of natural tooth jaw relationships.

  In clinical practice, complete denture treatment usually requires working casts to be articulated in centric relation (see below). The artificial tooth arrangement and jaw contact position between the denture teeth is then CO by definition.
- *Median occlusal position (MOP)* is a dynamic tooth contact position that may be determined by a 'snap' (rapid) jaw closure from a jaw open position (McNamara 1977). Tooth contacts at MOP have been proposed as being equivalent to functional tooth contacts. MOP tooth contacts can only be determined clinically and are useful to indicate functional tooth contacts in clinical occlusal analysis.

  The use of ultrafine occlusal tape (such as GHM Foil, Gebr. Hansel-Medizinal, Nurtingen, Germany; Ivoclar/Vivadent, Schaan, Liechtenstein), placed between the teeth (teeth need to be air-dried to allow the tape to mark tooth contacts), will allow MOP contacts to be identified.

  It is likely that MOP and ICP (with light tooth contact) are equivalent for clinical assessment purposes.
- *Retruded jaw position (RP)* is the position of the jaw when the condyles are in a physiologically acceptable guided position for the recording of transfer records. This position is a reproducible position for the treatment to be undertaken. It is not always constant in the long term, as remodelling adaptation of joint components is a feature of biological systems. RP is independent of tooth contacts.
- *Retruded contact position (RCP)* is the contact position of the teeth when the jaw is in RP.
- *Centric relation (CR)* is the jaw relationship (also termed maxillomandibular relationship) in which the condyles are located in an anterorsuperior position in contact with the central bearing surface (the thin avascular part) of the interarticular disc, against the articular eminence (Preston et al 1999) (Fig. 1.1). This position is independent of tooth contact.

  RP and CR are describing similar clinical anatomical relationships. It is the condylar position at RP or CR that is used for clinical recording of the jaw relationship for transfer to an articulator.
- *Postural jaw position (PJP)* is the position of the jaw when an individual is sitting or standing upright when relaxed and alert. There is variable space between

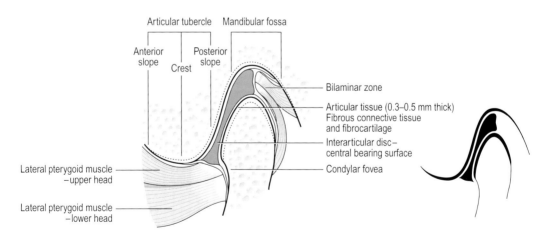

Fig. 1.1 Mid-sagittal section of the human temporomandibular joint. Note: (1) The extent of the central bearing surface of the interarticular disc. (2) The thickness of articular tissue varies, being thickest in those areas under greatest functional shear stress and load. This is illustrated in the lower right of the diagram where the surface tissues of the articulation are shown varying in thickness in the condyle, disc and temporal component. The dark areas represent the relative thicknesses, confirming that function occurs between condyle and articular tubercle rather than between condyle and fossa. (3) The anterior thick band (or foot) of the interarticular disc is bound down on the medial third to the superior surface of the superior lateral pterygoid muscle. Most muscle fibres insert into the condylar fovea. Some muscle fibres insert into a junctional zone between upper and lower heads, which then inserts into the fovea. More laterally, the anterior thick band attaches to the anterior capsular ligament.

maxillary and mandibular teeth, termed 'free-way' or speaking space. The PJP is determined by the weight of the jaw and the viscoelastic structural elements of the postural jaw muscles, as well as myotatic reflex contraction. This contraction is brought about by stretch of muscle spindles that results in activation of alpha-motoneurones that innervate the extrafusal muscle fibres of the jaw-closing muscles. PJP is important in the assessment of lower face height (lower third of the face as a proportion of overall facial proportion) and in determining the occlusal vertical dimension in treatment planning for dentate and edentulous patient needs.

- *Occlusal vertical dimension (OVD)* is the vertical height of the lower third of the face when the teeth contact in ICP. The lower third of the face is an important component of facial aesthetics and is an essential element of treatment planning in conjunction with PJP. The 'free-way' or speaking space is a variable separation of the teeth between PJP and OVD, and is an important determinant of speech communication. As a result, dental restorations may have a significant influence on speech in both dentate and edentulous treatment.
- *Lateral jaw positions*
  - *Mediotrusive* (or non-working or balancing) side refers to the side of the jaw which moves towards the midline (or medially) in lateral jaw movement. The term 'balancing' may also be understood in functional terms as the 'non-working' side, that is, the side opposite the chewing side.

    Non-working side is considered in the analysis of casts on an articulator, or the arrangement of the teeth for complete or partial dentures, in which non-working tooth contacts may be a desirable arrangement in denture construction. The term is also used in clinical occlusal analysis to identify the arrangement of teeth and the presence of mediotrusive (or balancing or non-working) tooth contacts or interferences (described in Chapter 5).
  - *Laterotrusive* (or working) side refers to the side of the jaw which moves laterally away from the midline in jaw movement. This may also be termed the 'working' or chewing side in function, that is, the side where chewing occurs.

    A particular aspect of laterotrusive jaw movement is the number and arrangement of the teeth which are in contact in lateral or laterotrusive jaw movement. This is also termed *disclusion*. Disclusion may involve the anterior teeth only, which may be the canine tooth (*canine disclusion*), or incisor and canine teeth (*anterior disclusion*); or it may involve posterior teeth only – bicuspid and/or molar teeth (*posterior disclusion*); or it may involve both anterior and posterior teeth (*group function*).

- *Bennett movement* and *Bennett angle* are terms originally described by Bennett (1906) as the first clinical study which identified lateral or sidewards movement of the jaw and differentiated the bilateral features of condyle movement with remarkable clarity in one subject (Bennett himself).
  - *Bennett movement* describes a lateral component of movement of the condyle with laterotrusive jaw movement. Bennett described a lateral horizontal component of movement, which has also been described in relation to the setting of articulator condylar guidance as 'immediate side shift' (ISS). The latter is strictly an articulator term. There is some evidence from clinical recordings (Gibbs & Lundeen 1982) that Bennett movement may occur in function, in some individuals, at the end of the closing path of a chewing movement.
  - *Bennett angle* is the angle formed by movement of the contralateral condyle with the sagittal plane during lateral jaw movement. The contralateral (or balancing) condyle moves downwards, forwards and medially, forming an angle (Bennett angle) with the sagittal plane when viewed anteriorly (from the front) or superiorly (from above).

    The articulator term for movement of the contralateral (or balancing) condyle is 'progressive side shift' (PSS).

OCCLUSAL RELATIONSHIPS

Confusion remains concerning optimum occlusal relationships and the association of occlusal variables with TMDs. In attempting to define what is optimum, it is acknowledged that stable occlusal relationships are the norm in the population, even though there is great variation in structural and functional features.

There are no controlled studies on the optimum features of a harmonious natural and/or restored occlusion. However, studies (Pullinger & Seligman 2000, Seligman & Pullinger 2000, Tsukiyama et al 2001) on the relationship between occlusal variables and TMDs provide a clue, even though there is a lack of agreement on this interrelationship (McNamara et al 1995, Kirveskari et al 1998).

Pullinger and Seligman (2000) and Seligman and Pullinger (2000) studied 12 independent variables together with age, and found that there was a significant overlap of occlusal features between asymptomatic control subjects and patients with TMDs. In general, their studies indicated that asymptomatic controls were characterised by:

- a small amount of anterior attrition
- small or no RCP – ICP slide (<1.75 mm)

- absence of extreme overjet (<5.25 mm), and
- absence of unilateral posterior crossbite.

However, sensitivity (61%) and specificity (51%) did not reach appropriately high enough levels (>75% and >90%, respectively) to provide undisputed evidence of association. In addition, McNamara et al (1995) reported that there is no link between changes in the occlusal scheme with orthodontic treatment and the development of TMDs.

In light of the information from these studies, it may be concluded that those occlusal features that are not associated with TMDs are acceptable as optimum for the individual. There are no doubt other features needing to be specified from research studies in order to more fully define optimum occlusion.

The recognition of a revised and limited role for occlusal variables in TMDs is significant, as it justifiably questions the historical emphasis given to the occlusion and its role in dysfunction.

In contrast with natural occlusions, in therapeutic restoration it is clinically desirable and practical, even in the absence of good research data, to optimise function by taking into account the following:

- Establish an appropriate occlusal vertical dimension for aesthetics (lower face height), functions of speech, mastication and swallowing, and to increase inter-occlusal space where necessary for restorations.
- Harmonise tooth contacts (maximum intercuspation) with a stable position of the condyles, ideally in an unstrained condylar position with interarticular discs appropriately aligned, to allow fluent function between condyle and eminence.
- The specific tooth contact pattern is not defined, but cusp–fossa and cusp–marginal ridge contacts provide stable tooth relationships; the need for tripodised contacts has not been established.
- Anterior tooth arrangement is crucial for aesthetics and speech. There is no evidence to support the need for either anterior guidance or group function (Marklund & Wänmann 2000, Yang et al 2000). However, in a consideration of the biomechanics of lateral tooth contact, anterior guidance makes sense, as bite force is reduced as well as the reaction force at the condyles. Smooth lateral and protrusive movements support fluent function, and may be important in optimising jaw muscle activity.

BORDER MOVEMENT

Posselt's border movement diagram

Posselt (1952) described the full range of jaw movement in three planes by tracing the path of the lower incisor teeth as the jaw is guided through the border paths. The

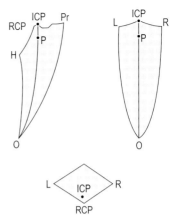

Fig. 1.2 **A** Shows the sagittal (or profile) view of the border diagram with the anteroposterior relationships of ICP, RCP and Pr. The view also shows that the lower incisor tooth movement from ICP to RCP requires the jaw to be guided into RCP. Lower incisor movement from RCP to H follows a curved path that reflects the initial rotatory movement of the condyles. This is also described as rotation around the intercondylar or terminal hinge axis, that is, the axis of rotation between the condyles when they are guided around centric relation. The movement changes from rotation to translation (H to O) after approximately 15–20 mm of jaw opening at the lower incisors. **B** Shows the frontal view and **C** the horizontal view of the movement of the lower incisors along the border path. The sagittal view is the most informative. ICP, intercuspal position; RCP, retruded contact position; Pr; protruded jaw position; P, postural jaw position; O, maximum jaw opening; H, hinge arc of opening. Approximate range of jaw movement in adults: RCP–ICP 0.5–2.0 mm; ICP–O 40–70 mm; RCP–H 15–20 mm; P–ICP 2–4 mm; ICP–Pr 5–10 mm.

border path is the maximum range of jaw movement which is determined by the jaw muscles, ligaments, movement limitations of the temporomandibular joints, and the teeth.

The teeth define the top of the border diagram which is of particular interest in restorative dentistry, as the relationship between ICP (IP) and CO (RCP) is diagrammatically indicated.

In the absence of teeth (as in complete edentulism) the top of the border diagram does not differentiate ICP (IP) and CO (RCP). The border diagram may be displayed in the sagittal, frontal and horizontal planes. The sagittal plane view of the border movement of the jaw in dentate individuals, as defined by the movement of the lower incisor teeth, shows features of particular interest:

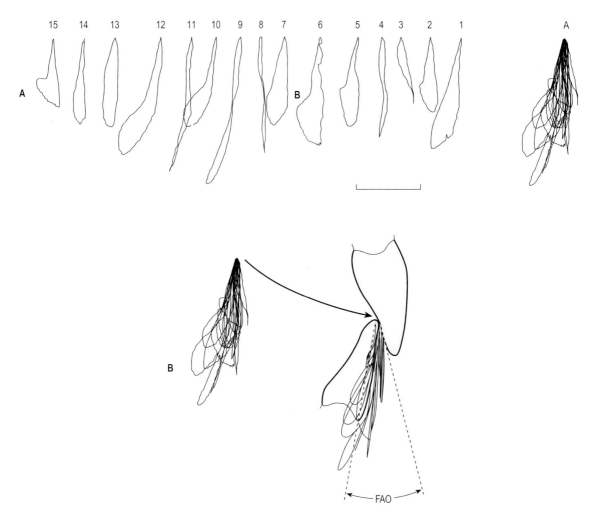

Fig. 1.3 **A** Tracings 1–15 represent individual chewing cycles (or envelopes) obtained by monitoring the movements of the lower incisor tooth while chewing gum. The movement of the lower incisor was recorded with a Kinesiograph (K5 Myo-tronics Research Inc., Seattle, Washington 98101, USA), via a magnet cemented at the incisors, and movement of the magnet was detected by an array of sensors (flux-gate magnetometers) attached to a headframe. Note the individual variations in each chewing cycle. The 15 cycles comprise the functional envelope of movement. (Bar indicates 10 mm.) **B** Tracings of the lower incisor tooth obtained as in **A** while chewing gum. The composite envelope of function is composed of the 15 individual chewing cycles shown in **A**. The relationship of the functional envelope to the incisor teeth is shown and the functional angle of occlusion (FAO) represents the approach and departure of the lower incisors from tooth contact.

- The top of the border path is defined by the position and cuspal inclines of the teeth (Fig. 1.2: ICP to RCP, ICP to Pr).
- The retruded path is defined by the anatomy of the temporomandibular joints (Fig. 1.2: RCP to H; H to O).

ANTERIOR OR LATERAL GUIDANCE

The physical features of tooth guidance vary with tooth arrangement and interarch relationships. Anterior guidance is provided by the vertical (overbite) and horizontal or anteroposterior (overjet) relationships of anterior teeth. Posterior guidance is determined by the relationships of supporting cusp inclines, particularly of opposing molar teeth. Posterior guidance may be increased in the presence of missing teeth, with tilting and drifting of teeth, and by the curvature of the occlusal plane anteroposteriorly (curve of Spee) and laterally (curve of Wilson). Tooth guidance varies between individuals and directly influences the approach and departure angle of mandibular to maxillary

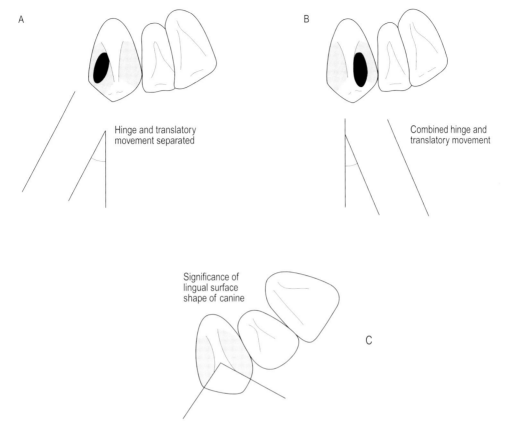

Fig. 1.4 Anterior guidance – functional angle of occlusion. **A** Anterior guidance on the distal incline of the ipsilateral canine tends to separate the distal hinge and translatory jaw movements, which may direct the condyle and disc along a more distal path and away from the eminence. **B** Anterior guidance on the mesial incline of the ipsilateral canine tooth tends to provide a combined hinge and translatory movement which may direct the condyle and disc along a more anterior path towards the eminence. **C** The lingual contour of the maxillary canine has a longitudinal ridge which divides the lingual surface into a distinct mesial and distal fossa. The opposing teeth (ideally the mandibular canine) may contact the distal or mesial fossa, and lateral jaw guidance will be different in each case. The distal fossa will tend to direct the jaw along a more distal (posterior) path and the mesial fossa will tend to direct the jaw along a more mesial (anterior) path.

teeth, that is, the functional angle of occlusion in chewing. The chewing cycle is also termed the envelope of function, the shape of which is determined by the tooth guidance (Fig. 1.3).

The functional loading of teeth and the associated stimulation of periodontal mechanoreceptors provide a reference point for tooth contact and establish a beginning and end of jaw movement in mastication and swallowing (Trulsson & Johansson 1996).

CANINE GUIDANCE

The lingual surface of the maxillary canine tooth is ideally contoured, with a prominent axial ridge that may provide mesial or distal guidance, depending on which surface the opposing tooth contacts. Lateral guidance on the distal canine surface may direct the ipsilateral (working) jaw distally, while initial tooth contact on the mesial canine incline may direct the jaw mesially. This may influence condyle disc relationships, although this has not been confirmed in clinical studies. This proposal is based on clinical and geometric assessment (Fig. 1.4).

Distal guidance

During function or parafunction, if anterior tooth guidance restricts the anterior component of movement (as is seen in the case of a deep bite), the closing jaw movement follows a more distal approach path to tooth contact. The more distal approach to tooth contact may also arise as a result of distal guidance from the canine that restricts forward translation in jaw closing. The more distally directed movement requires a predominance of condyle rotation. It is hypothesised that, with more rotation, the interarticular disc may more readily rotate beyond the posterior thick band of the disc and become trapped anteromedially. With translation, in contrast to rotation, the disc moves with the condyle, maintaining their relationship against the eminence.

Mesial guidance

Mesial guidance along the mesial canine incline may allow both rotation and translation. As a result, the jaw closes along a more anterior path and approaches tooth contact from a more forward position. It is hypothesised that this combination of rotation and translation encourages approximation of condyle interarticular disc with the posterior slope of the articular eminence, maintaining their contact relationships.

The association between mesial or distal canine guidance in lateral jaw movements, and the effect at the condyle, is complex and is linked with jaw muscle activity and condyle disc relationships. There is some clinical research evidence correlating distal canine guidance with a more posterior condylar path (Yang et al 2000). Yang et al described a weak correlation between distal canine guidance (that is, a retrusive laterotrusive path) and a lateral and posterior movement of the ipsilateral (working) condyle. In contrast, mesial canine guidance resulted in lateral and inferior movement of the ipsilateral condyle.

It is acknowledged that clinical studies to correlate jaw muscle activity with condyle disc relationships, to determine the influence of canine guidance, are difficult. The sophistication of equipment needed for accurately tracking condyle movement is a limitation, and the problem of identifying an appropriate point within the condyle for three-dimensional measurement has not been standardised (Peck et al 1999).

Although not necessarily a feature of the natural dentition, with clinical restoration of the dentition it is considered desirable to avoid mediotrusive (non-working) and laterotrusive (working) interferences (Wassell & Steele 1998, Becker et al 2000). The presence of guidance on canines is also preferred as a restorative convenience, although group function, where several teeth provide simultaneous lateral guidance, has been proposed to lead less readily to muscle fatigue (Møller & Bakke 1998).

A number of clinical physiological studies with electromyography and/or jaw tracking have attempted to determine the features of anterior guidance:

- Less muscle force is generated with anterior tooth contact only (Manns et al 1987), and maximum muscle force is developed with molar tooth contact; guidance from the anterior part of the jaw results in resolution of muscle force vectors to guide the jaw smoothly into IP.
- Belser and Hannam (1985) reported that:
  - There is no scientific evidence to indicate that canine guidance or group function is more desirable.
  - The steepness of the anterior guidance is not of primary importance.
  - The presence of a dominant canine guidance tends to reduce the opportunity for generating high interarch forces, and may reduce parafunctional loads.
  - Canine guidance does not significantly alter the masticatory stroke.
- Møller and colleagues (1988) have reported that:
  - Maximum occlusal stability and maximum elevator muscle activity occur at IP, suggesting that it is the optimum tooth contact position for chewing and swallowing.
  - Muscle activity is directly related to occlusal stability in ICP.
  - A critical relationship exists between contraction time and pause time in jaw-closing muscles and influences susceptibility to fatigue. Short, strong jaw-closing muscle contractions with a relatively long pause at tooth contact minimise the susceptibility to fatigue.
  - The relative contraction times of jaw-closing muscles in the chewing cycle were reduced in the presence of group function contacts for lateral guidance.
- More recently, Ogawa et al (1998) have reported that the chewing cycle is influenced by occlusal guidance and the occlusal plane inclination. Their studies were based on chewing gum and recording three-dimensional movement of jaw and condyle in relation to tooth guidance and occlusal plane orientation. They concluded that:
  - Both tooth guidance and occlusal plane orientation influence the form of the chewing cycle.
  - Occlusal guidance (overbite and overjet) influences the sagittal and frontal closing paths over the final 0.5 mm of jaw movement into tooth contact.
  - The occlusal plane angle influences the sagittal and frontal closing paths over the final 2.0–5.0 mm of jaw movement into tooth contact.

MEDIOTRUSIVE (BALANCING) CONTACTS/INTERFERENCES

Canine or anterior guidance is often present in the natural dentition of young individuals; however, tooth orientation in growth and development may result in posterior guidance. The variation in tooth arrangements and contact patterns in healthy adult dentitions is expected, linking form and function.

With tooth wear, group function develops as a feature of older natural dentition. In the process, mediotrusive contacts in lateral jaw movements may arise, as may mediotrusive interferences. A systematic review of the epidemiology of mediotrusive contacts by Marklund and Wänmann (2000) suggested a median percentage of the prevalence of mediotrusive contacts of 35% (studies reported 0–97%) and interferences of 16% (studies reported 0–77%). There were no gender differences. Steepness of the condylar inclination may influence the presence of mediotrusive contacts or interferences. This inclination changes with age and becomes steeper in adults. It follows that in children with flatter condylar inclinations there would be more mediotrusive interferences. This may be the case. However, the clinical significance is whether the presence of these contacts or interferences is associated with increased prevalence of jaw muscle pain and TMDs. There is some reported evidence that jaw muscle tenderness and impaired jaw movement is higher in children and young adults in association with mediotrusive interferences; however, the evidence is weak.

Research evidence suggests that:

- There is not a direct cause and effect relationship between posterior tooth contact relationship and either jaw muscle pain or TMDs (Clark et al 1999, Pullinger & Seligman 2000, Seligman & Pullinger 2000).
- Other factors are involved in the aetiology of TMDs.

A biomechanical study of mediotrusive contacts and clenching by Baba et al (2001) reported that canine guidance caused a small displacement at the ipsilateral molars and the largest displacement at the contralateral molars. A similar effect on condyle position is suggested, leading to limited compression of the ipsilateral joint and larger compression of the contralateral joint. It is possible that TM joint compression arising in this way may alter the biomechanical relationships of jaw muscles, condyle and disc and may be a predisposing factor or a possible initiating factor for TMDs.

EMG studies have confirmed specific changes in jaw muscles with mediotrusive and/or laterotrusive contacts, but no direct association with TMDs.

Recent studies on the influence of tooth contact interferences on jaw and joint position and jaw muscles suggest that:

- Specific changes in the occlusal scheme, such as placing mediotrusive (balancing) or laterotrusive (working) interferences, and canine guidance, cause predictable changes in jaw orientation (or tilt) with clenching (Minagi et al 1997, Baba et al 2001).
- Biomechanical associations occur as a result:

  – A mediotrusive interference and heavy bite force or clenching establish a lever arm with the interference as the fulcrum, leading to greater elevation of the ipsilateral molars and possible compression of the ipsilateral TM joint with a change in reaction force (Belser & Hannam 1985, Korioth & Hannam 1994, Baba et al 2001).

    It could be hypothesised that in some individuals parafunction in the presence of mediotrusive interferences and TM joint increased reaction force may contribute to TMD at the ipsilateral joint.

  – The presence of canine guidance eliminates mediotrusive interferences and changes the biomechanical effects of bite force and clenching on the TM joint.

    Baba et al (2001) showed that ipsilateral contact from canine to bicuspids to molars (that is, group function) with clenching leads to contralateral jaw elevation and joint compression. Canine guidance results in least joint compression, while ipsilateral molar contact interference with clench leads to greater contralateral joint compression. Such biomechanical changes with clenching may also be a possible contributing factor for TMD.

  – Balanced occlusion appears to be protective of the joints and may not lead to an increase in either ipsilateral or contralateral TM joint compression.

  – In support of the above, Minagi et al (1997) found a positive correlation between the absence of contralateral (mediotrusive) tooth contacts and increased prevalence of joint sounds. The corollary from this study is that mediotrusive contacts may have a protective role for the joint, in association with parafunction.

- In EMG studies, canine guidance results in increased unilateral anterior and posterior temporal activity. The presence of mediotrusive (balancing side) contacts recruits contralateral jaw muscles and results in bilateral anterior and posterior temporal activity (Belser & Hannam 1985, Baba et al 1996, Minagi et al 1997).

SHORTENED DENTAL ARCH (SDA)

It has been shown that individuals may have satisfactory aesthetics and occlusal function with a reduced number of posterior teeth (Käyser 2000). This fact has led to the so-called shortened dental arch concept and the realisation that it is not always necessary to replace missing posterior teeth.

Of particular interest in the management of the occlusion is the recognition of the concept of the shortened dental arch as a viable treatment option. This section concerns specific tooth contact relationships and the controversial effects of clenching on the TM joints and describes studies based on the presence of posterior (bicuspid and molar) teeth.

In the absence of the molar and possibly bicuspid teeth, the specific lever arm effects and TM joint reaction forces from loading would not occur to the same extent. Whether or not this is advantageous to the jaw muscle system would depend on remaining tooth distribution and their ability to withstand functional and parafunctional loading.

More importantly, the often claimed association between the lack of posterior teeth predisposing to TM joint loading and the possible development of TMD is not supported. Long-term data on the clinical effects of the shortened dental arch indicates that the absence of molar teeth does not predispose to TMD or orofacial pain, and allows adequate function for long-term health of the jaw muscle system.

The minimum number of teeth needed for function varies with individuals. The goal of maintaining a complete dental arch, although theoretically desirable, may not be attainable or necessary. It has been shown from long-term studies that the anterior and premolar segments can meet all functional requirements (Käyser 2000).

When priorities have to be set, restorative treatment should preserve the most strategic anterior and premolar segments. The need for partial dentures or complex treatment to restore molar segments (implant, bridgework, endodontics and root/tooth resection) should be questioned and based on individual patient wishes.

References

Baba K, Yugami K, Yaka T, Ai M 2001 Impact of balancing-side tooth contact on clenching-induced mandibular displacement in humans. Journal of Oral Rehabilitation 28:721–727

Becker C M, Kaiser D A, Schwalm C 2000 Mandibular centricity: centric relation. Journal of Prosthetic Dentistry 83:158–160

Belser U C, Hannam A G 1985 The influence of altering working-side occlusal guidance on masticatory muscles and related jaw movement. Journal of Prosthetic Dentistry 53:406–414

Clark G T, Tsukiyama Y, Baba K, Watanabe T 1999 Sixty-eight years of experimental interference studies: what have we learned? Journal of Prosthetic Dentistry 82:704–713

Forssell H, Kalso E, Koskela P et al 1999 Occlusal treatments in temporomandibular disorders: a qualitative systematic review of randomised controlled trials. Pain 83:549–560

Gibbs C H, Lundeen H C 1982 Jaw movements and forces during chewing and swallowing and their clinical significance. In: Lundeen H C, Gibbs C H (eds) Advances in occlusion. Wright, Boston, pp 2–32

Käyser A F 2000 Limited treatment goals – shortened dental arches. Periodontology 4:7–14

Kirveskari P, Jamsa T, Alanen P 1998 Occlusal adjustment and the incidence of demand for temporomandibular disorder treatment. Journal of Prosthetic Dentistry 79:433–438

Korioth T W, Hannam A G 1994 Mandibular forces during simulated tooth clenching. Journal of Orofacial Pain 8:178–189

McNamara D C 1977 The clinical significance of median occlusal position. Journal of Oral Rehabilitation 5:173–186

McNamara J A, Seligman D A, Okeson J P 1995 Occlusion, orthodontic treatment and temporomandibular disorders. A review. Journal of Orofacial Pain 9:73–90

Manns A, Chan C, Miralles R 1987 Influence of group function and canine guidance on electromyographic activity of elevator muscles. Journal of Prosthetic Dentistry 57:494–501

Marklund S, Wänmann A 2000 A century of controversy regarding the benefit or detriment of occlusal contacts on the mediotrusive side. Journal of Oral Rehabilitation 27:553–562

Minagi G, Ohtsuki H, Sato T, Ishii A 1997 Effect of balancing-side occlusion on the ipsilateral TMJ dynamics under clenching. Journal of Oral Rehabilitation 24:57–62

Møller E, Bakke M 1988 Occlusal harmony and disharmony: frauds in clinical dentistry. International Dental Journal 38:7–18

Ogawa T, Koyano K, Umemoto G 1998 Inclination of the occlusal plane and occlusal guidance as contributing factors in mastication. Journal of Dentistry 26: 641–647

Peck C C, Murray G M, Johnson C W L, Klineberg I J 1999 Trajectories of condylar points during working-side excursive movements of the mandible. Journal of Prosthetic Dentistry 81:444–452

Posselt U 1952 Studies in the mobility of the human mandible. Acta Odontologica Scandinavica 10:1–160

Preston J D, Blatterfein L, South F 1999 Glossary of prosthodontic terms. Journal of Prosthetic Dentistry 81:39–110

Pullinger A G, Seligman D A 2000 Quantification and validation of predictive values of occlusal variables in temporomandibular disorders using a multi-factorial analysis. Journal of Prosthetic Dentistry 83:66–75

Riise C, Ericsson S G 1983 A clinical study of the distribution of occlusal tooth contacts in the intercuspal position in light and hard pressure in adults. Journal of Oral Rehabilitation 10:473–480

Seligman D A, Pullinger A G 2000 Analysis of occlusal variables, dental attrition, and age for distinguishing healthy controls from female patients with intra capsular temporomandibular disorders. Journal of Prosthetic Dentistry 83:76–82

Trulsson M, Johansson R S 1996 Encoding of tooth loads by human periodontal afferents and their role in jaw motor control. Progressive Neurobiology 49:267–284

Tsukiyama Y, Baba K, Clark G T 2001 An evidence-based assessment of occlusal adjustment as a treatment for temporomandibular disorders. Journal of Prosthetic Dentistry 86:57–66

Wassell R W, Steele J G 1998 Considerations when planning occlusal rehabilitation: a review of the literature. International Dental Journal 48:571–581

Yang Y, Yatabe M, Ai M, Soneda K 2000 The relation of canine guidance with laterotrusive movements at the incisal point and the working-side condyle. Journal of Oral Rehabilitation 27:911–917

2 Jaw movement and its control

G. Murray

Synopsis

The jaw muscles move the jaw in a complex three-dimensional manner during jaw movements. There are three jaw-closing muscles (masseter, temporalis and medial pterygoid) and two jaw-opening muscles (lateral pterygoid and digastric). The basic functional unit of muscle is the motor unit. The internal architecture of the jaw muscles is complex, with many exhibiting a complex pennate (feather-like) internal architecture. Within each of the jaw muscles the central nervous system (CNS) appears capable of activating separate compartments with specific directions of muscle fibres. This means that each jaw muscle is capable of generating a range of force vectors (magnitude and direction) required for a particular jaw movement.

The CNS activates single motor units in whatever muscles are required to generate the desired movement. Movements are classified into voluntary, reflex and rhythmical. Many parts of the CNS participate in the generation of jaw movements. The face motor cortex is the final output pathway from the cerebral cortex for the generation of voluntary movements. Reflexes demonstrate pathways that aid in the refinement of a movement and can also be used by the higher motor centres for the generation of more complex movements.

Mastication or chewing is a rhythmical movement that is controlled by a central pattern generator (CPG) in the brainstem. The CPG can be modified by sensory information from the food bolus and by voluntary will from higher centres. Simple jaw movements can also be performed, such as protrusion and side-to-side movements. At any instant in time, the jaw can be described as rotating around an instantaneous centre of rotation.

Many devices have been constructed to describe jaw movements but only six-degrees-of-freedom devices can accurately describe the complexity of movement. The use of devices that provide single point tracings (for example, pantographs) may provide misleading information if used for diagnostic purposes or in the evaluation of treatment outcomes. Masticatory movements are complex and consist of jaw, face and tongue movements that are driven by jaw, face and tongue muscles. Changes to the occlusion appear capable of having significant effects on the activity of the jaw muscles and the movement of the jaw joint.

Key points

- The jaw muscles move the jaw in a complex three-dimensional manner
- There are three jaw-closing muscles (masseter, temporalis and medial pterygoid) and two jaw-opening muscles (lateral pterygoid and digastric)
- The functional unit of muscle is the motor unit
- The internal architecture of the jaw muscles is highly complex
- Jaw muscles generate a range of force vectors (magnitude and direction) required for a particular jaw movement
- The CNS activates motor units in whatever muscles are required to generate the desired movement
- Movements are classified into voluntary, reflex and rhythmical
- Many parts of the CNS participate in the generation of jaw movements

- Reflexes demonstrate a pathway that can be used by the higher motor centres for the generation of more complex movements
- Mastication is controlled by a central pattern generator in the brainstem
- At any instant in time, the jaw can be described as rotating around an instantaneous centre of rotation
- The use of devices that provide single point tracings (for example, pantographs) may provide misleading information if used for diagnostic purposes or in the evaluation of treatment outcomes
- Changes to the occlusion appear capable of having significant effects on the activity of the jaw muscles and the movement of the jaw joint

JAW MUSCLES: THE MOTORS FOR JAW MOVEMENT (for reviews, see Hannam & McMillan 1994, van Eijden & Turkawski 2001)

An understanding of jaw movement provides background for Chapter 8 on jaw muscle disorders, which describes changes in jaw movement patterns.

- There are three jaw-closing muscles: masseter, temporalis and medial pterygoid.
- There are two jaw-opening muscles: digastric and lateral pterygoid.
- The contractile element of muscles is the motor unit. Each motor unit consists of an alpha-motoneurone plus all the muscle fibres (~600–1000) innervated by (that is, connected to and activated by) that motoneurone. Jaw muscle motoneurones are mostly located in the trigeminal motor nucleus.
- There are three physiological types of motor units that contribute to variations in the magnitude of force that different motor units generate. Type S motor units are slow, generate low forces and are fatigue resistant. Type FF motor units are fast, generate the highest forces but fatigue rapidly. Type FR motor units have intermediate speed and force generating capabilities, and have intermediate fatigue resistance. Type S motor units are recruited first in a muscle contraction. With larger forces, Type FR and then type FF motor units are recruited.
- Further complexity is added by the fact that each face, jaw or tongue muscle has a complex internal architecture in terms of the arrangement of the muscle fibres within each muscle. The masseter muscle, for example, contains muscle fibres arranged in a pennate manner (that is, a feather-like arrangement). Figure 2.1 illustrates some of the aponeurotic sheaths dividing the

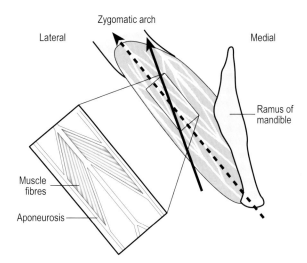

Fig. 2.1 Coronal view through the masseter muscle, zygomatic arch and ramus of mandible. Some of the aponeuroses that divide up the masseter have been outlined and are shown in expanded form on the left. The feather-like (pennate) arrangement of the muscle fibres is indicated by the heavy lines. The solid arrow demonstrates the direction of pull if the labelled muscle fibres were to selectively contract. The dashed arrow indicates the direction of pull if the muscle fibres hypothetically passed directly from the zygomatic arch to the mandible.

masseter. An expanded view of part of the muscle (left of figure) shows the pennate arrangement of muscle fibres (heavy lines). When motor units on one side of the aponeurosis contract, they direct forces at an angle (the pennation angle) to the long axis of the muscle and generate a force vector (that is, magnitude and direction of force) at an angle (solid arrow in Figure 2.1) to the force vector that would be generated if muscle fibres passed directly from the zygomatic arch to the ramus without pennation (dashed arrow). These complexities of muscle fibre architecture provide a wide range of directions with which forces can be applied to the jaw. The brain can selectively activate these regions, or subcompartments, independently of other regions of the muscle.

- When generating a particular movement of the jaw, the sensorimotor cortical regions that drive voluntary movements (see below) are not organised in terms of specific muscles to activate. Rather, they send a command signal to the various motor nuclei to activate those motor units, in whatever muscles are available, that are biomechanically best suited to generate the force vector required for that particular jaw movement. Thus, for example, a grinding movement of the jaw to the right side with the teeth together might be best achieved by activation of some motor units in the inferior head of the left lateral pterygoid, some motor units in the right posterior temporalis to prevent the right side of the jaw moving forwards, and some units in the right masseter and anterior temporalis to help pull the jaw to the right side and to keep the teeth together while doing so (Miller 1991). The activation of these motor units will produce a force on the jaw that moves the jaw to the right side.

CNS COMPONENTS IN THE GENERATION AND CONTROL OF JAW MOVEMENTS (Fig. 2.2)

- Motor cortex and descending pathways through pyramidal tract to alpha-motoneurones (drives motor units).
- Cerebellum (refinement and co-ordination of the movement).
- Basal ganglia (selects and initiates motor programmes).
- Supplementary motor area (SMA), premotor cortex (area 6) (contains programmes for movements).
- Central pattern generators for mastication and swallowing (programmes for generating mastication and swallowing).

Some important connections of the orofacial motor system

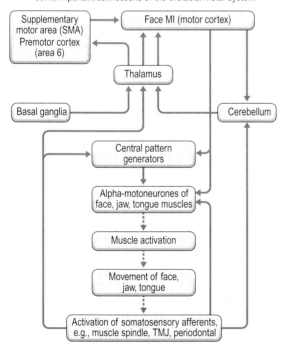

Fig. 2.2 Some important connections of the orofacial motor system. Arrows indicate some of the complex linkages in the sequence leading to a motor event. Solid arrows indicate direction of action potentials conveying information. Dotted arrows indicate the result of an event.

- Alpha-motoneurones within brainstem motor nuclei.
- Motor units within muscles.
- Somatosensory system that conveys and processes somatosensory information about the movement.

CLASSIFICATION OF JAW MOVEMENTS

- Voluntary movements: for example, playing the piano, speaking, taking an alginate impression, moving the jaw forwards.
- Reflex movements: for example, knee-jerk reflex, jaw-jerk reflex, jaw-opening reflex.
- Rhythmical movements: for example, chewing, walking, running, breathing.

Voluntary movements (for review, see Hannam & Sessle 1994)

- Voluntary movements are driven by the primary motor cortex (termed MI) and higher motor cortical areas (supplementary motor area (SMA), premotor cortex).
- When patients are asked to move the tongue forwards and open the jaw (as when taking an impression), a set of programmes (much like computer programs) is selected and activated (via the basal ganglia) and these programmes send signals to the MI, specifically the face region. They contain the details of those motor units that must be activated, and the sequence of activation, to produce a particular movement. The programmes probably reside in the SMA/premotor cortical regions. The MI is responsible for activating the various motor units to produce the movement required.
- The face MI consists of specific output zones within the cerebral cortex that send fibres in the pyramidal tract to synapse directly or indirectly (via interneurones) onto alpha-motoneurones. Each output zone from the face MI activates a specific elemental movement; for example, movement of the tongue forwards or movement of the tongue to the side, or elevation of the corner of the mouth, or jaw opening or jaw movement to the side. The same movement can be produced at a number of different sites throughout the face MI.
- The face MI can be considered to be the 'keys of a piano' that the higher motor centres 'play' to allow the generation of the required voluntary movement. Combinations of output zones allow the generation of more complex movements (equivalent to the generation of more complex sounds, as when playing chords on a piano).
- The cerebellum continuously coordinates movements by controlling the sensory inputs to the motor areas.
- Corrections to each movement can also occur via shorter pathways that involve fewer neurones and many of these pathways are located entirely at the brainstem level. These pathways can be demonstrated clinically by evoking reflexes.

Reflex movements (for review, see Hannam & Sessle 1994)

• Reflex movements are largely organised at the brainstem or spinal cord level. They are stereotyped movements that are involuntary and are little modified by voluntary will.

• The classic reflex is the knee-jerk reflex where a sharp tap to the knee evokes contraction in the thigh muscles and a brief lifting of the lower leg.

• Other reflexes are the *jaw-closing* or *jaw-jerk reflex*, and the *jaw-opening reflex*.

• The jaw-closing reflex occurs when the jaw-closing muscles are suddenly stretched by a rapid downwards tap on the chin. This tap causes stretching of specialised sensory receptors called muscle spindles that are stretch-sensitive. They are present within all the jaw-closing muscles. When spindles are stretched, a burst of action potentials travel along the group Ia primary afferent nerve fibres coming from the primary endings within the

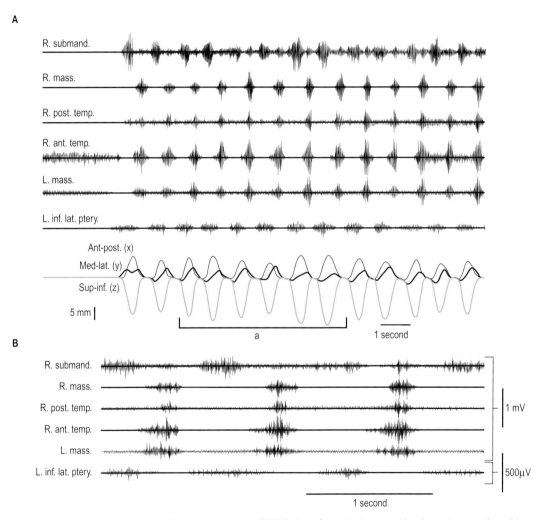

Fig. 2.3 Right-sided gum chewing. **A** Electromyographic (EMG) data from six jaw muscles (top six traces) and jaw movement data (bottom three traces) during 13 cycles of chewing of gum. The EMG activity was recorded from the submandibular group of muscles (R. submand.; principally the anterior belly of the digastric muscle), the right and left masseter (R. mass., L. mass.), the right posterior temporalis (R. post. temp.), the right anterior temporalis (R. ant. temp.), and the left inferior head of the lateral pterygoid (L. inf. lat. ptery.) muscles. The movement traces display the movement of the midincisor point of the mandible in anteroposterior (Ant-post.), mediolateral (Med-lat.) and superoinferior (Sup-inf.) axes. Thus, for example, the latter shows the amount of vertical displacement of the midincisor point during the opening phase of each chewing cycle. **B** Expanded form of the EMG data only from the section labelled 'a' in **A**.

spindles. The primary afferents synapse directly onto and cause activation of the alpha-motoneurones of the same jaw-closing muscle. Thus a stretch of a jaw-closing muscle leads to a fast contraction of the same jaw-closing muscle.

- Reflexes demonstrate a pathway that can be used by the higher motor centres for the generation of more complex movements. They also allow fast feedback that adjusts a movement to overcome small, unpredicted irregularities in the ongoing movement and adds smoothness to a movement.

- The jaw-opening reflex can be evoked by a variety of types of orofacial afferents. Activity in orofacial afferents, for example, from mucosal mechanoreceptors, passes along primary afferent nerve fibres to contact inhibitory interneurones that then synapse on jaw-closing alpha-motoneurones. The inhibitory interneurones reduce the activity of the jaw-closing motoneurones. At the same time, primary afferents activate other interneurones that are excitatory to jaw-opening muscles, such as the digastric. The overall effect is an opening of the jaw.

Rhythmical movements (for reviews, see Lund 1991, Hannam & Sessle 1994)

- These movements share features of both voluntary and reflex movements. The reflex features of rhythmical movements arise because we do not have to think about these movements for them to occur. For example, we can chew, breathe, swallow and walk without thinking specifically about the task; however, we can at any time voluntarily alter the rate and magnitude of these movements.

- Rhythmical movements are generated and controlled by collections of neurones in the brainstem or spinal cord. Each collection is called a *central pattern generator* (CPG). The CPG for mastication is located in the pontine–medullary reticular formation. Figure 2.2 shows some relations of the CPGs. Swallowing is not a rhythmical movement but it is also controlled by a CPG located in the medulla oblongata.

- The CPG is essentially equivalent to a computer program. When activated, the CPG for mastication, for example, sends out appropriately timed impulses of the

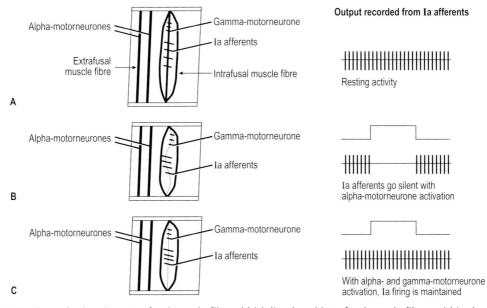

Fig. 2.4 Stylised muscle showing extrafusal muscle fibres (thick lines) and intrafusal muscle fibres within the muscle spindle under three conditions. **A** The resting condition, where, in this hypothetical muscle, there is a resting tension on the muscle which comes from, for example, the weight of the mandible at postural jaw position. The slight stretch to the muscle from the weight of the mandible results in a slight stretching of the intrafusal muscle fibres and group Ia afferent terminals that results in a continuous barrage of action potentials passing centrally. **B** In the hypothetical situation where only alpha-motoneurones are firing, muscle fibres contract and this results in a reduced tension in the muscle spindle and therefore the spindle Ia afferent firing ceases for the duration of the contraction. During this period, the spindle is unable to provide information about unexpected changes in muscle length. **C** Shows alpha-motoneurone activation accompanied by gamma-motoneurone activation (alpha-gamma coactivation – the usual situation in any movement) so that the intrafusal muscle fibres contract at the same rate as the extrafusal muscle fibres. This maintains the tension at the terminals of the Ia afferents so that they maintain their firing and are able to respond to, and signal irregularities in, the movement.

appropriate magnitude to the various jaw, face and tongue muscle motoneurones so that the rhythmical movement of mastication can occur. We do not have to think about what muscles to activate and the relative timing of activation of the muscles in order to carry out mastication. This is done by the CPG. We can, however, voluntarily start, stop and change the rate and magnitude and shape of the chewing movements, and these modifications are done through descending commands to the CPGs from the motor cortical regions.

• Figure 2.3A shows raw electromyographic (EMG) data from a number of jaw muscles during right-sided chewing of gum. The associated movement of the mid-incisor point is shown in the lower part. Note the regular bursting pattern of EMG activity that occurs in association with each cycle of movement. Note also, in the expanded version in Figure 2.3B, that the EMG activity from the inferior head of the lateral pterygoid muscle and the submandibular group of muscles is out of phase with the jaw-closing muscles. These muscles are being controlled by the CPG, and many other jaw, face and tongue muscles, not recorded here, are being activated similarly.

• Sensory feedback is provided by mechanoreceptors located within orofacial tissues: for example, periodontal (that signal magnitude and direction of tooth contact), mucosal (that signal food contact with mucosa), muscle spindle (that signal muscle length and rate of change of muscle length as the jaw closes), Golgi tendon organ (that signal forces generated within muscles) and temporomandibular joint (TM joint) (that signal jaw position) mechanoreceptors.

• The muscle spindle is a very complicated sensory receptor. Muscle spindle sensitivity is optimised for all lengths of a muscle. During a muscle contraction, both alpha- and gamma-motoneurones are activated. The alpha-motoneurones cause contraction of the main (extrafusal) muscle fibres and are responsible for the force produced by muscles (Fig. 2.4A, B). The gamma-motoneurones are activated at the same time but they cause contraction of the intrafusal muscle fibres within the muscle spindle and thus maintain the sensitivity of the spindles as the muscle and spindles shorten (Fig. 2.4C). The spindle is therefore always able to detect small changes in muscle length irrespective of the length of the muscle.

• Sensory information plays a crucial role in modifying mastication (for review, see Lund & Olsson 1983). During chewing, there is a huge barrage of sensory information that travels into the CNS (Fig. 2.5A). Some of this information travels directly to the cerebral cortex for conscious sensation (Fig. 2.2).

– Local reflex effects that assist the masticatory process also occur. For example, as food is crushed between the teeth, periodontal mechanoreceptors are activated, and this activity can cause a reflex *increase* in activity

in the jaw-closing muscles to assist in crushing of food.

– Many of the orofacial afferents that are activated by food contact during jaw closing can evoke a jaw-opening reflex (see above). This would be counter-productive during the closing phase of mastication. Lund and Olsson (1983) have shown that the masticatory CPG depresses the responsiveness of the jaw-opening reflex during the closing phase of the chewing cycle. The low T (that is, threshold) test reflex response shown in Figure 2.5B on the far left is the control jaw-opening reflex response, seen in the digastric muscle, to the activation of orofacial afferents when there is no chewing. During the closing phase of the chewing cycle, the CPG depresses the ability to evoke this reflex. Therefore, in chewing, the excitatory pathway from orofacial afferents to jaw-opening motoneurones is depressed, and this allows the jaw to close unhindered.

– An analogous effect occurs during the opening phase of the chewing cycle. During this phase, muscle spindles in jaw-closing muscles will be stretched and will have a tonic excitatory effect on jaw-closing motor units. This would resist jaw opening. However, the CPG hyperpolarises jaw-closing motoneurones during the opening phase of the chewing cycle (Fig. 2.5B). This hyperpolarisation makes jawclosing moto-neurones harder to activate in response to excitatory input from muscle spindles.

BASIC MANDIBULAR MOVEMENTS

• The jaw can be viewed as being suspended from the skull by muscles, tendons, ligaments, vessels and nerves and is moved in three-dimensional space, with the fixed points being the teeth and the condyles in their respective condylar fossae.

• Basic mandibular movements are open, close, right-side jaw movement, left-side jaw movement, protrusion, retrusion.

• Factors influencing mandibular movements:

– condylar guidance: the inclination of the pathway travelled by the condyle during a protrusive or a contralateral jaw movement; these two inclinations will usually be slightly different

– incisal guidance: determined by anterior tooth relationships, that is, the magnitude of overbite (vertical overlap) and overjet (horizontal overlap) between anterior teeth

– posterior guidance: determined by posterior tooth relationships

– muscles and ligaments.

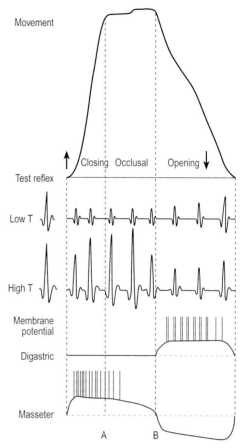

A Afferent firing

Movement

Muscle and receptor activity

Closing | Occlusal | Opening

Opener EMG

Closer EMG

Peridontal RA / SA

Cutaneous RA / SA

M spindle 1° / 2°

A   B

B Reflex modulation

Movement

Test reflex

Low T

High T

Membrane potential

Digastric

Masseter

A   B

Fig. 2.5   A Some of the patterns of jaw muscle and somatosensory afferent activity during masticatory jaw movements. The movement of the jaw at the midincisor point is at the top. The next two traces show jaw-opener and jaw-closer EMG activity, respectively. Periodontal and cutaneous mechanoreceptive activity are shown next. RA, rapidly adapting, that is, responds only to the dynamic phases of, in this case, a mechanical stimulus; SA, slowly adapting, that is, responds to dynamic and static components of a mechanical stimulus. M spindle 1°, 2°, refers to output from muscle spindle group Ia (provides information on dynamic changes in muscle length), and group II (provides information on new muscle lengths) primary afferents, respectively. Each vertical line in each trace shows the time of occurrence of an action potential that has been recorded in the primary afferent axon. There is a barrage of sensory information that enters the brain during every chewing cycle. **B** The jaw-opening reflex is modulated during mastication. The left shows the type of reflex response that is recorded from the digastric muscle with the jaw at rest (control). Note that the amplitude of this reflex changes during mastication. When low-threshold afferents are stimulated (low T, that is, non-painful), the mean amplitude is less, especially during the closing and occlusal phases. In contrast, the response to high-threshold afferents (high T) exceeds the control during the late closing and occlusal phases. This pathway is facilitated during the closing phase of the chewing cycle – it is desirable to stop the closing phase of chewing should painful stimuli be encountered during this phase. The lower two traces show that the digastric membrane is at its resting level during these phases, and masseteric motoneurones are hyperpolarised during the opening phase to reduce the possibility of these motoneurones firing, particularly under the influence of group Ia and II muscle spindle afferent barrage arising because muscle spindles are being stretched during the opening phase. (Adapted with permission.)

- Movements to and from intercuspal position. Of interest to clinicians are:
  - group function: defined as an occlusion in which the occlusal load in lateral excursion is distributed across at least two pairs of teeth on the working side
  - mutually protected (~10% of natural dentitions) (or canine-guided) occlusion: only the anterior (or canine) teeth are in contact in any excursive movement of the jaw.
- Mastication is not a simple open–close jaw movement. Because the condyles are able to translate forwards as

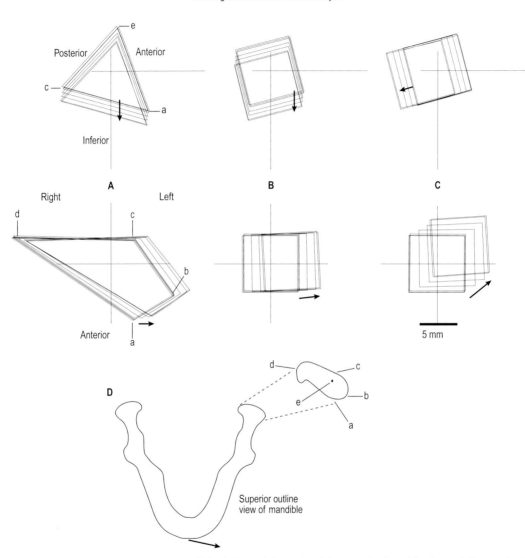

Working side movement of left condyle

Fig. 2.6 Detail of working side movement of the left condyle. Sagittal (upper plots) and horizontal (lower plots) plane views of condylar triangles (upper plots in **A**) and quadrilaterals (lower plots in **A**) for the left condyle in a subject performing a working-side mandibular movement, that is, the jaw moves to the left side. A superior view of mandible is shown in **D** and the condylar points are labelled: a, anterior; b, lateral; c, posterior; d, medial; e, superior (this point was 9.0 mm superior to the other points). The points were determined from computer tomography scans of the subject. **B** shows sagittal (upper) and horizontal (lower) squares generated about the origin of the respective axes in **A**. **C** shows sagittal and horizontal squares generated about an origin that was shifted 30 mm further laterally. A square, triangle or quadrilateral is plotted each 300 ms, starting at the intercuspal position. In each trace, the outgoing movement only is shown from intercuspal position to maximum lateral excursion and the approximate direction of movement is indicated by a short arrow. The trajectories of individual condylar points have been omitted for clarity. (Adapted with permission.)

well as rotate, there are constantly changing combinations of rotation and translation during mastication.

• Instantaneous centre of rotation of the jaw. At any instant in time, the jaw can be described as rotating around a centre of rotation. This centre of rotation is constantly shifting because of constantly changing combinations of translation and rotation during most jaw movements.

– A protrusive jaw movement with sliding tooth contact consists largely of translation of the jaw forwards, with a slight downwards translation. With a steeper incisal than condylar guidance, the jaw will also rotate open slightly. The instantaneous centres of rotation will lie well below and posterior to the jaw.

– For a left-side jaw movement with sliding tooth contact, most of the movement is rotation about a constantly moving centre of rotation lying in the vicinity of (usually behind and lateral to) the left condyle. Figure 2.6A shows sagittal (upper plots) and horizontal (lower plots) plane views of condylar triangles (upper plots in A) and quadrilaterals (lower plots in A) for the left condyle in a subject performing a working-side mandibular movement, that is, the jaw moves to the left side. The quadrilaterals are formed by joining the points a, b, c and d on the actual outline of the condyle in the horizontal plane shown in Fig. 2.6D. The triangles are formed by joining the points a, e and c on the condyle; point e is a point 9 mm superior to the other points. A triangle or quadrilateral is plotted each 300 ms from intercuspal position (IP). During this working-side movement in the horizontal plane, the condyle does *not* rotate about the centre of the condyle but rather the centre of rotation can be visualised to be behind the condyle.

– At each successive instant in time during chewing, the centre of rotation shifts in space. For chewing jaw movements, this centre lies between the lower posterior parts of the jaw and towards the midline.

HOW TO DESCRIBE JAW MOVEMENT?

• For over a century, dentists have had a keen interest in the movement of the jaw and have attempted to describe its movement by graphical devices such as pantographs and more sophisticated jaw-tracking devices. One of the reasons for doing this has been to make it easier to perform restorative work for patients.

• These systems usually record the movement of the anterior midline of the lower jaw (for example, see Figure 2.3) or the terminal hinge axis or the palpated lateral condylar pole in three degrees of freedom, that is, the movement of a single point along anteroposterior, mediolateral and superoinferior axes (Fig. 2.3). They do not provide information about the three rotation vectors:

pitch, yaw and roll. This additional information is provided by six-degrees-of-freedom systems.

• It has been recently shown that considerable error is introduced to the pathway that condylar-point tracings follow simply because of the selection of a different point in the vicinity of the condyle (Peck et al 1997, 1999). Thus, many of the irregularities in condylar-point tracings that have been ascribed diagnostic or prognostic significance could simply have occurred because of the location of the condylar point chosen. Figure 2.6B shows the movement of points chosen at equal distances about the coordinate centre in Figure 2.6A. The resulting squares move in a similar fashion to the quadrilaterals and triangles in A. Figure 2.6C shows the effect on the movement recorded simply by shifting the points 30 mm laterally. The interpretation of the movement of the condyle plotted in C would be that the condyle has translated posteriorly and laterally, whereas in fact the condyle has largely translated laterally with some rotation.

• Single point tracings may therefore provide misleading information if used for diagnostic purposes or in the evaluation of treatment outcomes.

• Border movements of the jaw are described in Chapter 1.

MASTICATORY JAW MOVEMENTS
(Lund 1991)

• Masticatory jaw movements occur well within these border movements except when the jaw approaches or makes tooth contact towards the end of chewing.

• In the frontal plane, the masticatory cycle is classically described as 'tear-drop' in shape. At the beginning of opening, the mid-incisor point moves first downwards and at the end of opening it moves laterally and upwards towards the working side (or chewing side). The mid-incisor point then moves upwards and medially and the food is crushed between the teeth.

• The masticatory sequence is highly variable from cycle to cycle in a subject chewing the same or different foods and from subject to subject. Figure 2.3A (lowermost traces) shows that the movement of the midincisor point from cycle to cycle is not identical. Part of this variability relates to the changing consistency of the food bolus from cycle to cycle as the food breaks down. The movement of the jaw towards IP is less variable. The jaw muscles must move the jaw precisely towards the end of the chewing cycle, so that the teeth glide smoothly along cuspal inclines. Mechanoreceptors (particularly periodontal) provide a continual source of afferent input to the CNS to ensure the chewing cycle is harmonious with existing tooth guidances (Ch. 1).

• Masticatory movements are complex and consist of jaw, face and tongue movements that are driven by jaw, face and tongue muscles. The facial and tongue muscles are involved because the lips, cheeks and tongue help control the food bolus in the mouth and keep the food contained over the occlusal table for effective comminution.

• It is remarkable that the tongue is largely made of the very substance that the teeth commonly break down. The author believes that the face MI strongly inhibits jaw-closing muscles before any tongue movements are allowed to occur. The tongue is most active during the opening phase of the chewing cycle when food is required to be collected and repositioned for effective comminution on the occlusal table.

• Different phases of masticatory cycles:
- preparatory phase: jaw, tongue, lips and cheeks prepare the bolus for effective food comminution
- reduction phase: period of food comminution associated with salivary flow and mix of food and saliva
- preswallowing: food is brought together as a bolus with saliva, which commences the chemical breakdown process, and is prepared for swallowing.

• The shape and duration of the cycle is influenced by the hardness of food: harder textured foods are associated with wider chewing cycles that have longer duration. Softer foods are associated with more up and down chewing cycles (Gibbs & Lundeen 1982).

CONDYLE AND DISC MOVEMENT

• The movement of the condyle and disc during normal jaw movements is complex and not well understood (Scapino 1997). The issue is complicated by the fact that the lateral pterygoid muscle inserts into the TM joint, with the inferior head inserting exclusively into the condylar neck and the superior head inserting largely into the condylar neck.

• Some fibres of the superior head do insert into the disc–capsule complex of the TM joint, but the long-held view (still held by some) that the superior head inserts exclusively into the disc is completely erroneous! Further, the view that the superior and inferior heads of the lateral pterygoid muscle exhibit reciprocal patterns of activity is also erroneous. Our research group has recently proposed that the superior head (and the inferior head) of the muscle is actually like multiple smaller muscles, each able to be independently activated and thus able to provide the appropriate force vector onto the condyle and disc–capsule complex to produce the movement required.

• Do changes to the occlusion have any influence on the movement of the jaw and the jaw joint? Our research group has also recently proposed that this is so and the implication of these data is that whatever we do to the occlusion can have significant effects on jaw and jaw-joint movement and the function of the jaw muscles. Recent data suggest that the placement of an occlusal interference results in a decrease in activity in most of the jaw muscles, except the lateral pterygoid muscle, where an increase in activity may be observed.

• Thus, restoring teeth, in such a way that results in interferences with the normal pathways of a chewing cycle, can lead to different levels of firing of orofacial afferents (for example, periodontal afferents). This information will feed back to the CNS and may cause a change to the CPG controlling mastication, or to higher levels of the CNS, for example, face MI. This change will be in the form of changes to the firing of particular motor units, in particular subcompartments of muscles, so that the appropriate modification to the chewing cycle can occur. The new chewing cycle will now avoid this interference unless the interference is too large and beyond the adaptive capacity of the CPG and muscles.

References

Gibbs C H, Lundeen H C 1982 Jaw movements and forces during chewing and swallowing and their clinical significance. In: Lundeen H C, Gibbs C H (eds) Advances in occlusion. Wright, Boston, pp 2–32

Hannam A G, McMillan A S 1994 Internal organization in the human jaw muscles. Critical Reviews in Oral Biology and Medicine 5:55–89

Hannam A G, Sessle B J 1994 Temporomandibular neurosensory and neuromuscular physiology. In: Zarb G A, Carlsson G E, Sessle B J, Mohl N D (eds) Temporomandibular joint and masticatory muscle disorders. Munksgaard, Copenhagen, pp 80–100

Lund J P 1991 Mastication and its control by the brain stem. Critical Reviews in Oral Biology and Medicine 2:33–64

Lund J P, Olsson K A 1983 The importance of reflexes and their control during jaw movement. Trends in Neurosciences 6:458–463

Miller A J 1991 Craniomandibular muscles: their role in function and form. CRC Press, Boca Raton

Peck C, Murray G M, Johnson C W L, Klineberg I J 1997 The variability of condylar point pathways in open–close jaw movements. Journal of Prosthetic Dentistry 77:394–404

Peck C, Murray G M, Johnson C W L, Klineberg I J 1999 Trajectories of condylar points during working-side excursive movements of the mandible. Journal of Prosthetic Dentistry 81:444–452

Scapino R P 1997 Morphology and mechanism of the jaw joint. In: McNeill C (ed) Science and practice of occlusion. Quintessence, Chicago, pp 23–40

van Eijden T M G J, Turkawski S J J 2001 Morphology and physiology of masticatory muscle motor units. Critical Reviews in Oral Biology and Medicine 12:76–91

3 Growth and development

J. Knox

Synopsis

Three-dimensional skeletal proportions are the primary determinant of the relationship between maxillary and mandibular dental arches. An appreciation of craniofacial growth and development is, therefore, essential in the understanding of the aetiology of normal and abnormal static and functional occlusal relationships.

   More detailed descriptions of pre- and postnatal craniofacial development are available elsewhere (Bjork 1968, Enlow 1982). This chapter will provide an overview of dentofacial development, focusing on how normal variation and abnormal growth and development can influence intra- and interarch relationships.

Key points

- Skeletal relationships at birth
  - Prenatal events
- Normal skeletal development
  - Maxilla
  - Maxilla relative to cranium
  - Mandible
  - Mandible relative to cranium and maxilla
    Growth rotations
  - Timing
  - Prediction
- Normal dental development
  - Timing
  - Space considerations
  - Interarch relationships
- Abnormal skeletal development
  - Aetiology
  - Anteroposterior
  - Transverse
  - Vertical
- Abnormal dental development
  - Aetiology
  - Interarch relationships
  - Arch length discrepancies
  - Local factors
- Late changes
  - Skeletal
  - Dental
- Orthodontic solutions

NORMAL SKELETAL DEVELOPMENT

The craniofacial relationships present at birth are a product of rapid cell multiplication, differentiation and migration. The cranial vault is composed of frontal, parietal, squamous temporal and occipital bones. These bones are formed by intramembranous ossification and are separated by relatively loose connective tissues that allow cranial deformation during birth. In contrast, the bones of the base of the skull are formed initially in cartilage. Centres of endochondral ossification appear early in embryonic life, indicating the ultimate location of the basioccipital, sphenoid and ethmoid bones that form the cranial base. As ossification proceeds, bands of cartilage remain as spheno-occipital, sphenoethmoidal and intersphenoidal synchondroses.

   The maxilla develops essentially as a membranous bone from infraorbital centres of ossification with a small contribution from partial cartilaginous ossification of the nasal capsule. From these centres, frontal, zygomatic, alveolar and palatal areas develop. The mandible is formed, similarly, by intramembranous ossification in fibrocellular condensations alongside Meckel's cartilage and the inferior dental nerve, and ossification of the secondary condylar cartilage.

   Postnatal facial growth and development is classically described as a downward and forward displacement of the maxillary complex and mandible relative to the cranial base, involving a process of sutural responses to functional skeletal displacements and surface remodelling.

Apposition of bone at the periphery of the cranial bones rapidly reduces the volume of interposed connective tissue, resulting in the bones being separated by thin periosteum-lined sutures. It is the apposition of bone at these sutures that provides the major mechanism for growth of the cranial vault, with remodelling of the inner and outer surfaces of the bones providing the means by which recontouring occurs.

In the cranial base, cellular proliferation at the sphenoethmoidal synchondrosis is responsible for growth of the anterior cranial base until its fusion at about 7 years. The spheno-occipital synchondrosis remains patent until the late teen years and contributes to growth of the posterior cranial base and anterior displacement of the midface.

Growth of the maxilla occurs by surface remodelling and by apposition of bone at the sutures that connect the maxilla to the cranium and cranial base. During normal facial growth the maxilla is translated downward and forward. During this translation bone is laid down in the tuberosity region and at the sutural attachments of the maxilla to the cranial vault and base, increasing the size of the bone and maintaining sutural dimensions. Interestingly, as the maxilla is translated forward and downward, the anterior surface of the bone is remodelled and bone is removed, resulting in a change in contour due to periosteal activity.

During normal growth, the mandible is also translated downward and forward relative to the cranial base. However, in contrast to the maxilla, both endochondral and periosteal activity are important in the growth of the mandible. Vital staining experiments have shown that bone is primarily deposited on the posterior surfaces of the ramus, coronoid process and condyle, while bone resorption occurs on the anterior ramal surface and chin as the mandible is translated forward in its soft tissue envelope.

CHANGE IN RELATIVE PROPORTIONS

The pattern of postnatal growth results in a change in proportions so that the head, which at birth contributes 30% of the total body length, in adulthood contributes only 12%. The advanced development of the cranial and uppermost structures of the body relative to more proximal areas is suggested to represent a 'cephalocaudal gradient of growth'. This gradient is seen in craniofacial development, with the cranial vault being relatively large at birth and the face small and retrusive. Postnatal growth changes these proportions and the midface becomes less retrusive, with the mandible being the last of the facial bones to finish anteroposterior development.

In addition to downward and forward translation of the maxilla and mandible described, longitudinal cephalometric implant studies (Bjork 1968) have demonstrated that there is a rotation of the central core of these bones, the magnitude of which is masked by surface changes and tooth eruption (Bjork & Skeiller 1983). For an average individual, the net change during growth is a slight reduction in lower facial height. However, for patients with longer or shorter faces than average, the amount of core (internal) rotation and surface change can vary, resulting in significant alterations in vertical facial proportions, interarch relationships and incisor inclinations during growth.

The rate of craniofacial growth is greatest during the first years of life. Thereafter, other than for the small prepubertal and more significant pubertal growth 'spurts', the rate of growth and change in proportions decline to almost zero by 16–18 years of age. It would be incorrect to assume that growth and change in facial proportions ceases in adulthood. Longitudinal cephalometric evaluation of adults involved in the Bolton growth study (Broadbent et al 1975) has demonstrated that cumulative changes occurring in both facial dimensions and proportions continued up to the age of 35–40 years, resulting in altered incisor inclinations and vertical interarch relationships.

NORMAL DENTAL DEVELOPMENT

Tooth eruption

When a tooth emerges into the mouth, it has a *postemergent spurt* and erupts rapidly until it approaches the occlusal plane and is subject to the forces of mastication. Eruption then slows dramatically as the period of *juvenile occlusal equilibrium* is reached. During this period, teeth that are in function erupt at a rate that parallels the rate of vertical growth of the mandibular ramus. This is best appreciated by considering the relative submergence of ankylosed teeth during growth.

During the pubertal growth, there is a further increase in tooth eruption as the interocclusal space is increased. It would appear that the forces that oppose a tooth's eruption, such as occlusal forces and the forces generated by resting soft tissues, are the rate-limiting factors in postemergent eruption rather than the eruptive forces themselves. At the end of this *circumpubertal eruptive spurt* an *adult occlusal equilibrium* is reached in which tooth eruption may compensate for occlusal wear.

Eruption of the primary dentition

The timing of eruption of the primary dentition is variable and up to 6 months of acceleration or delay is within the

Table 3.1 Eruption of primary dentition

	Calcification begins (weeks in utero)	Crown complete (months)	Eruption (months)
Incisors	13–16	1.5–3.0	6–9
Canines	15–18	9	18–20
First molars	14–17	6	12–15
Second molars	16–23	10–11	24–36

normal range. The eruption sequence is, however, usually preserved and most commonly the mandibular central incisor erupts first, closely followed by the other incisors.

Three to four months later, the mandibular and maxillary first molars erupt, followed by the maxillary and mandibular canines 3–4 months after that. The primary dentition is usually complete by 24–30 months when the second molars erupt (Table 3.1).

Spacing is normal throughout the anterior part of the primary dentition but is most noticeable in the primate spaces that lie between canine and lateral incisor in the maxilla and between canine and first molar in the mandible. Generalised spacing of the deciduous teeth is a requirement for correct alignment of the permanent labial segment.

Mixed dentition years

The mixed dentition years include dental ages 6–12. Dental age is determined by the teeth that have erupted, the root development of the permanent teeth and the degree of resorption of the primary teeth. The transition from the primary to the permanent dentition begins at about 6 years with the eruption of the first permanent molars, followed soon thereafter by the permanent incisors.

Dental age 7 is characterised by eruption of maxillary central incisors and mandibular lateral incisors. The root development of the maxillary lateral incisor is advanced at this stage and the canines and premolars are completing crown formation. Dental age 8 is characterised by the eruption of the maxillary lateral incisor and is followed by a period of 2–3 years before any other permanent teeth erupt.

There are significant space considerations during the replacement of the deciduous incisors, as each of the permanent incisors is 2–3 mm larger than its predecessor. Spacing of the primary dentition will usually provide sufficient space to accommodate the larger central incisors and often the lateral incisors, in the upper arch. In the mandible, however, there is on average 1.6 mm less space available than that required for perfect alignment of the lower four permanent incisors. This space discrepancy, called the 'incisor liability', often results in a transitory stage of mandibular incisor crowding at age 8–9 years that remains until eruption of the canines.

The larger permanent incisors are therefore accommodated by using the primate spaces and generalised labial segment spacing. In addition, the permanent intercanine width is increased and the incisors erupt in a more proclined relationship which places them on the arc of a larger circle. It is important to note that all of these changes occur without significant growth at the front of the jaws.

A widely recognised developmental stage, which not infrequently causes parental concern, is the midline diastema and distal inclination of the maxillary central incisors. The spacing seen in this 'ugly duckling' stage will invariably reduce as the lateral incisors erupt but may persist if the primary canines have been lost or the incisors are flared labially. As a rule of thumb, a diastema of 2 mm or less will probably close spontaneously when the permanent canines erupt, whereas the diastema may persist when the original dimensions exceed 2 mm.

At dental age 9 the root development of mandibular canines and first premolars is 30% complete and the second premolar has started root formation. In the maxilla, however, development is not as advanced and only the first premolar has started root formation.

By dental age 10 the root development of upper canine and upper and lower second premolar is more significant and the roots of the lower canine and upper and lower first premolars are 50% complete. The roots of the incisor teeth are virtually complete at this stage and the resorption of primary canines and molars is more advanced.

At dental age 11–12 the remaining succedaneous teeth erupt and the final phases of the establishment of the permanent dentition begin. The space requirements during the replacement of the primary canines and molars are extremely important. In contrast to the anterior teeth, the premolars are smaller than the teeth that they replace. The result is a 'leeway space' of 1.5 mm per quadrant in the maxillary arch, while the space in the mandibular arch measures 2.5 mm per quadrant.

The interarch relationship of the first permanent molars during the mixed dentition period would be classified by Angle as half a unit class II, that is, there is a flush terminal plane. The correction of this molar relationship to class I, in the development of normal occlusion, requires that the lower molar move forward by 3.5 mm relative to the upper. Approximately half of this distance is provided by the differential anteroposterior growth of the mandible during this period and the remainder is provided by the greater mandibular leeway space.

Establishment of the secondary dentition

Following the eruption of the second permanent molars at 12–13 years, the permanent dentition is virtually complete, leaving only the third molars to erupt at 18–21 years. However, the dentition established during the teenage years often changes significantly during the late teens and early twenties. Reduction in the size of pulp chambers, apical migration of periodontal attachment and a degree of occlusal and interproximal wear have been recorded as normal maturational changes in the dental apparatus. In addition, more recent longitudinal studies (Sinclair & Little 1985) have recorded significant changes in dental alignment with time, particularly in the mandibular labial segment.

There have been a number of theories proposed to account for the increased lower incisor irregularity with age. Pressure from erupting third molars has been suggested as a likely cause, mainly due to the coincidence of third molar eruption with late lower incisor imbrication. The force generated by erupting teeth is, however, only 5–10 g and late lower incisor crowding has been recorded in individuals who have congenitally absent third molars and in those who have had the third molars removed at a young age (Vasir & Robinson 1991, Harradine et al 1998).

The reduced interproximal attrition associated with modern diets has been suggested to have a possible aetiologic role in the development of late lower incisor crowding, as have alterations in the tone of facial musculature and mesially directed forces of occlusion. However, contemporary thought considers late incisor crowding to be the result of continued anteroposterior and rotational growth of the mandible during early adult life. Therefore, patients who have had ideal alignment of their labial segments during their early teens, whether due to orthodontic treatment or not, will not infrequently present with a variable degree of lower incisor imbrication during later life (Sinclair & Little 1985).

AETIOLOGY OF MALOCCLUSION

An important concept in the study of growth and development is variability. A large amount of the available information is derived from cross-sectional studies in which the samples have sometimes been selected on the basis of normal facial proportions and interarch relationships (Riolo et al 1974, Broadbent et al 1975).

The incidence of malocclusion varies depending on the age and race of the sample and the method of assessment employed. In most instances, malocclusion and dentofacial deformity result not from some pathological process but from moderate distortions of normal development. Skeletal disproportion can occur in any of the three dimensions, resulting in anteroposterior, vertical and transverse discrepancies and, depending on the degree of dentoalveolar compensation, abnormal intra- and interarch tooth relationships.

Dentoalveolar factors include those conditions in which there is a discrepancy between the sum of the mesiodistal widths of the teeth present in an arch and the space available for the teeth (arch length discrepancies) and a number of abnormalities that affect an isolated area of dental development (local factors).

Aetiology of skeletal disproportion

The determinants of craniofacial growth have been suggested to be the bone itself, the cartilaginous components and the soft tissue matrix in which the skeletal elements are embedded. The major difference in the theories is the location at which genetic control is expressed and contemporary thought would suggest that the truth lies in some synthesis of the second and third theories, that is, growth is determined by cartilaginous and soft tissue elements.

The response of sutures and periosteal tissues to transplant experiments and environmental influences suggests that these tissues are not primary determinants of growth but instead add or remove bone in response to bony displacement. Similar animal experiments suggest that the mandibular condyle is not a growth centre and instead behaves more like a reactive periosteal surface. The cartilage of the nasal septum, however, has been suggested to be a pacemaker for other aspects of maxillary growth and loss of this cartilage has been seen to result in a maxillary hypoplasia.

The functional matrix theory (Moss & Sanlentijn 1969) suggests that the growth of the face occurs as a response to functional needs and is mediated by the soft tissues in which the jaws are embedded. Growth of the cranium illustrates this theory well. Growth of the brain results in expansion and separation of the bones of the cranial vault, which in turn leads to sutural deposition of bone and increased cranial volume. When applied to the growth of the maxilla and mandible, this theory suggests that enlargement of the nasal and oral cavity in response to functional demands results in displacement and growth of the facial skeleton. In favour of this theory is the reduced growth observed where function is impeded, such as the mandibular hypoplasia associated with condylar ankylosis.

The aetiology of a number of skeletal discrepancies is well established. Congenital dentofacial anomalies, condylar hyperplasia and skeletal disproportion due to trauma are good examples. The remainder of the skeletal discrepancies are due to a combination of genetic and environmental factors.

Genetic influences on the development of skeletal disproportion have been evaluated by 'outbreeding' studies and comparison of monozygotic twins. Cross-breeding between genetically different human subgroups could result in the inheritance of discordant dental and facial characteristics. In the early 1970s studies were performed on the effects of outbreeding on the indigenous Polynesian population of the Hawaiian Islands following the influx of Caucasian and Oriental settlers. They found that the prevalence of extreme jaw relationships in the offspring of the various racial crosses was similar to that of the ancestral groups. However, there were some additive effects, that is, if the ancestral Polynesian population had 10% crowding, while the Japanese group had 10% class III, there would be approximately a 10% incidence of both characteristics in the offspring.

The fact that dental and facial characteristics are not inherited as clearly discernible single gene effects does not mean that there is not a strong hereditary component in the development of dental and facial proportions. Similar facial proportions and occlusal traits have been noted in family members but these similarities could be due to a common environment. Differences between genetically identical monozygotic twins can only be accounted for by environmental influences. Some twin studies have concluded that 50% of occlusal variations could be accounted for on the basis of heritability, leaving 50% due to environmental influences. However, others argue that if appropriate corrections for similar environment are made, the estimate for heritability drops almost to zero.

When considering the functional influences on skeletal growth, mouth breathing has been in and out of vogue as a possible aetiological factor of malocclusion. Respiratory needs are the primary determinant of jaw and head posture and it has been proposed that mouth breathing, by altering these postures, can affect both jaw growth and tooth position.

Humans are primarily nasal breathers, but transition to partial oral breathing occurs at elevated ventilatory exchange rates or increased nasal resistance levels. Chronic nasal obstruction results in a lowering of the mandible, downward and forward positioning of the tongue and a tipping back of the head. The type of malocclusion associated with mouth breathing is called 'long face syndrome' and its features are:

- downward and backward mandibular rotation during growth
- excessive eruption of posterior teeth
- a tendency towards maxillary constriction
- excessive overjet
- anterior open bite.

However, the relationship between mouth breathing, altered posture and the development of malocclusion is not clear-cut. Mouth breathing, in short, can undoubtedly contribute to the development of orthodontic problems, exaggerating existing tendencies for skeletal discrepancy, but partial nasal obstruction is difficult to indict as a major aetiological agent.

Dentoalveolar factors

When the aetiology of arch length discrepancies and local factors is considered, genetic influences may be evaluated by considering the extent to which malocclusion was present in early humans as compared to its prevalence under modern conditions. Crowding and malalignment were not unknown in prehistoric times but the overall perspective is that the prevalence of malocclusion has increased in modern times. There are two possible explanations for this increase on genetic grounds. The first is the additive effect of outbreeding, as discussed earlier; the second is the tendency for evolutionary reduction in jaw size.

It can be appreciated that there would be a tendency for crowding and malalignment to develop if the rate of reduction of jaw size were faster than the reduction of tooth size or number. The difficulty with this theory is that the increase in the prevalence of malocclusion has occurred too rapidly during the last few hundred years, whereas evolutionary drift, if this occurs, would take place over a longer time scale.

In addition to skeletal disproportion and arch length discrepancies, a number of local disturbances of dental development may play an important role in the development of a malocclusion. Significant disturbances include:

- abnormalities of tooth number
- abnormalities of tooth size and shape
- interference with eruption
- ectopic eruption
- improper guidance of eruption
- early loss of primary teeth
- premature loss of permanent teeth
- soft tissue factors.

Abnormalities of tooth number

Congenital absence of teeth results from disturbances during the initiation and proliferation of tooth formation. Anodontia or oligodontia, the absence of all or most teeth, is often associated with ectodermal dysplasia, but oligodontia may occur in a patient with no apparent systemic problem or congenital syndrome. Anodontia and oligodontia are rare, but hypodontia is a relatively common finding with a prevalence of 1.5–3.0%, depending on the sample.

Absence of a deciduous tooth is quite rare but when it occurs the upper 'B' is most commonly affected. The permanent teeth most commonly missing are upper lateral incisors, lower second premolars, third molars and, less commonly, lower central incisors.

Supernumerary teeth result from disturbances during the initiation and proliferation stages of dental development. Supernumerary teeth occur most frequently near the upper midline somewhat palatal to the central incisors, in the lower premolar region, and distal to the second and third molars. Supernumeraries in the premolar and molar regions generally have little effect on the teeth of the normal series but rotation or delayed eruption of a central incisor, or a large permanent diastema, may accompany a supernumerary in the incisor region.

Abnormalities of tooth size and shape

Abnormalities of tooth size and shape result from disturbances during the morphodifferentiation stage of development. The most common abnormality is a variation in size, particularly of maxillary lateral incisors and second premolars.

About 5% of the total population has a significant 'tooth size discrepancy' because of disproportionate sizes of upper and lower teeth. Occasionally, tooth buds may fuse or geminate during their development, making the development of normal occlusion impossible.

Interference with eruption

Delays in eruption of permanent teeth contribute to malocclusion, primarily because other teeth drift to undesirable positions in the arch. In 10–15% of children, at least one primary molar becomes ankylosed before it finally resorbs and exfoliates. This delays the eruption of its successor and malocclusion will result if drift or tilting of surrounding teeth occurs.

Occasionally, malposition of a permanent tooth bud can lead to ectopic eruption. The teeth most likely to be affected are the maxillary first molars, incisors and canines. If the eruption path of the maxillary first molar carries it too far mesially, impaction against the distal root of the second primary molar, with subsequent loss of this tooth, will result in a reduction of arch length and malocclusion. Ectopic eruption of mandibular lateral incisors, which occurs more frequently than first molars, may lead to transposition of the lateral incisor and canine. Ectopic eruption has been implicated in the aetiology of the impacted maxillary canine but other considerations, including arch length discrepancies and physical obstruction of eruption, may contribute to this tooth's impaction.

Improper guidance of eruption

At one time, the space closure accompanying early loss of primary teeth was attributed entirely to mesial drift of posterior teeth, which was confidently ascribed to forces from occlusion. The contemporary view is that mesial drift is inhibited by, rather than caused by, occlusal forces. However, whatever the cause, mesial drift of the first permanent molar after a primary second molar is prematurely lost can contribute significantly to posterior arch crowding.

Following the premature loss of a primary first molar or canine, space closure results primarily from distal drift of the incisors due to trans-septal fibre contraction and cheek/lip pressure. Unilateral loss of a primary canine or first molar will lead to an asymmetry of the occlusion and a tendency toward crowding.

Dental trauma

Dental trauma can lead to the development of malocclusion in three ways:

- damage to permanent tooth buds from an injury to the primary teeth
- drift of permanent teeth after premature loss of primary or permanent teeth
- direct injury to permanent teeth.

Trauma to a *primary tooth* that displaces an underlying permanent tooth bud can result in defective amelogenesis of the permanent tooth, if enamel formation is occurring at the time of the injury, or displacement of the crown relative to its root, if crown formation is complete. Root formation may stop, leaving a permanently shortened root or, more frequently, root formation continues at an angle to the displaced crown, resulting in dilaceration. If distortion of the root position is severe enough, it is almost impossible for the crown to assume its correct occlusal position.

Traumatic avulsion of *primary* incisors is unlikely to lead to significant drift of permanent teeth, but early avulsion is likely to delay the eruption of the permanent successors due to the slow resorption of the layer of compact bone that forms in the edentulous area. If a permanent incisor is avulsed at an early age, drift of the other permanent teeth may result in an unsightly space too small for adequate prosthetic replacement. If a posterior tooth is lost prematurely to trauma, the same patterns of drift will occur as if it had been lost to caries (see later).

Soft-tissue factors

The forces contributing to the equilibrium position of the dentition are masticatory forces, eruptive forces, and the forces exerted by the lips, cheeks and tongue. Although one might think that force magnitude and duration would determine the biological response of the dentition, it has been shown that the force duration is by far the most important consideration, and that heavy intermittent pressures, such as those exerted by masticatory muscles, have little impact on the long-term position of a tooth (Proffit 1978). Indeed, very light forces are successful in moving teeth, if the force is of long enough duration. The duration threshold seems to be approximately 6 hours in humans, a duration exceeded by the lips, cheeks and tongue at rest. It seems unlikely that the intermittent short-duration pressures, generated when the tongue and lips contact the teeth during swallowing or speech, would have any significant impact on tooth position.

Another possible contributor to the dental equilibrium is the periodontal fibre system. A contribution to horizontal equilibrium is made by the trans-septal fibres, as seen by the tendency of orthodontically moved teeth to return toward their pretreatment positions, and a contribution to vertical equilibrium is made by the tooth's eruptive force, which opposes the intrusive vectors of soft tissue resting pressures. In the absence of space created by extraction or orthodontic tooth movement, the gingival fibre network apparently has minimal effects on the horizontal dental equilibrium. However, the vertical equilibrium of the dentition is an important consideration in the aetiology of malocclusion related to function.

Although almost all normal children engage in non-nutritive sucking, prolonged sucking habits can lead to malocclusion if they persist into the mixed dentition years. The malocclusion results from a combination of direct pressure on the teeth and an alteration in the pattern of resting cheek and lip pressures, and is characterised by flared maxillary incisors, proclined or retroclined lower incisors, anterior open bite and a constricted maxillary arch. Direct pressure from the digit is presumably responsible for incisor displacement, while interference with normal labial segment eruption and excessive buccal segment eruption are responsible for the anterior open bite. The constricted maxillary arch results from the lowered tongue posture and disruption of the force equilibrium experienced by the maxillary posterior teeth.

In summary, the simple clear-cut explanations of malocclusion on a primary genetic basis that were widely accepted in the past have been demonstrated to be incorrect. Skeletal and dentoalveolar orthodontic problems can arise from inherited patterns, defects of embryological development and trauma, with a variable contribution made by other functional influences. The majority of patients presenting with malocclusion do so because of a genetic predisposition to their condition, an environmental influence that altered their ideal pattern of development, or some combination of genetic predisposition exaggerated by environmental influences.

The management of malocclusion commonly involves orthodontic, operative and sometimes surgical specialities to normalise intra- and interarch relationships by tooth movement, dentofacial orthopaedics and restorative care.

References

Bjork A 1968 The use of metallic implants in the study of facial growth in children: method and application. American Journal of Physical Anthropology 29:243–250

Bjork A, Skeiller V 1983 Normal and abnormal growth of the mandible: a synthesis of longitudinal cephalometric implant studies over a period of 25 years. European Journal of Orthodontics 5:1–46

Broadbent B H Sr, Broadbent B H Jr, Golden W H 1975 Bolton standards of dentofacial developmental growth. Mosby, St Louis

Enlow D H 1982 Handbook of facial growth. W B Saunders, Philadelphia

Harradine N W, Pearson M H, Toth B 1998 The effect of extraction of third molars on late lower incisor crowding: a randomised controlled trial. British Journal of Orthodontics 25:117–122

Moss M, Sanlentijn L 1969 The primary role of functional matrices in facial growth. American Journal of Dentofacial Orthopedics 55:566–577

Proffit W R 1978 Equilibrium theory revisited. Angle Orthodontist 48:175–186

Riolo M L, Moyers R E, McNamara J A, Hunter W S 1974 An atlas of craniofacial growth. Monograph 2, Craniofacial, growth series, University of Michigan, Ann Arbor

Sinclair P, Little R M 1985 Dentofacial maturation in untreated normals. American Journal of Orthodontics 85:146–156

Vasir N S, Robinson R J 1991 The mandibular third molar and late crowding of the mandibular incisors – a review. British Journal of Orthodontics 18:59–66

Further reading

Proffit W R, Fields H W 2000 Contemporary orthodontics. Mosby, St Louis, chapters 2–5

4 Anatomy and pathophysiology of the temporomandibular joint

S. Palla

Synopsis

The temporomandibular (TM) joint is a freely movable articulation between the mandibular condyle and the glenoid fossa, with the articular disc interposed. Movements occur by a combination of rotation (between condyle and disc) and translation (between the condyle–disc complex and the fossa). This high degree of mobility, in particular of the translatory movement, is reflected in the way in which the disc is attached to the condyle and in the absence of hyaline cartilage. Condyle and fossa are covered by fibrocartilage and the disc consists of a dense collagen fibre network oriented in different directions related to functional load.

Condylar movements are complex, and during chewing both condyles are loaded, the working less than the non-working condyle. The TM joint is able to adapt to load changes by remodelling. TM joint osteoarthrosis is a primarily non-inflammatory joint disease characterised by destruction of the cartilage and exposure of the subchondral bone. Central to the osteoarthrotic process is the production of proteolytic enzymes by chondrocytes. Progression is probably determined by the joint-loading condition.

This chapter is an overview of the anatomy, the histology of the articular disc and its attachments to the condyle and fossa, condylar movements, joint remodelling and joint osteoarthrosis.

Key points

- Temporomandibular joint anatomy
  - Temporal component
  - Mandibular condyle
  - Articular disc
  - Joint capsule
  - Disc attachments
  - Disc position
  - Joint innervation
  - Joint lubrication
- Condylar movements
  - Rotation versus translation
- Joint loading
- Joint remodelling
  - Disc remodelling
- Joint osteoarthrosis

TEMPOROMANDIBULAR JOINT ANATOMY

The temporomandibular (TM) joint is a freely movable articulation between the condyle of the mandible and the glenoid fossa – part of the squamous portion of the temporal bone. In comparison to other body articulations this joint has some unique features:

- Functionally the TM joint is a bilateral joint – the right and left joint always function together.
- The condyle–disc complex has a high degree of mobility and condylar movements always occur by a combination of rotation and translation. Thus, the TM joint is classified as a ginglymodiarthroidal joint, that is, a joint in which both rotatory and gliding (translatory) movements take place.
- The articulating surfaces are not covered by hyaline but by fibrocartilage.
- Condylar movements are controlled not only by the shape of the articulating surfaces and the contraction patterns of the muscles but also by the dentition. The

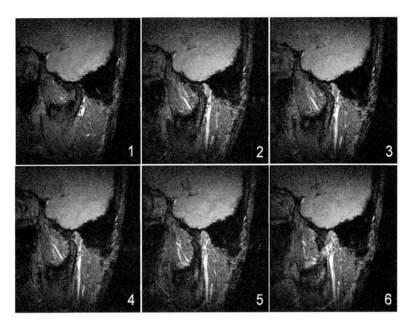

Fig. 4.1 Six positions of the condyle–disc complex during an opening movement. While the condyle rotates below the disc, the condyle–disc complex glides anteriorly. Note that at maximum opening the disc lies on top of the posterior part of the condylar head.

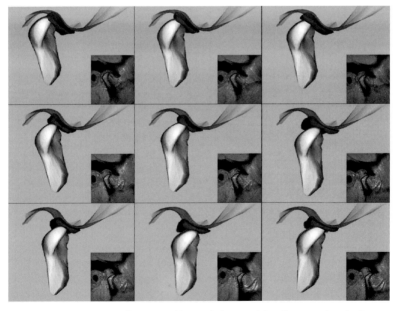

Fig. 4.2 Three-dimensional reconstruction of nine positions of the condyle–disc complex during an opening movement. Note that the condyle–disc complex translates less anteriorly than in the sequence shown in Fig. 4.1. As a consequence the degree of rotation of the condyle is less.

dentition also determines the end position as well as the movement of the condyle–disc complex when jaw movements are performed with the teeth in contact, as at the end of chewing or during tooth grinding.

Condyle and fossa are separated by the articular disc, which is attached to both condyle and fossa by means of disc attachments. The condyle articulates against the disc, forming the condyle–disc complex, which articulates with

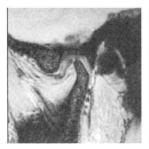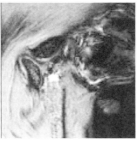

A   B

Fig. 4.3 Magnetic resonance image of disc position in maximum intercuspation (**A**) and at maximum opening (**B**). At maximum intercuspation, the condyle lies behind the disc, whereas at maximum opening it is normally positioned below the disc (for comparison, see Fig. 4.1). In order to reach this position the condyle translates below the disc.

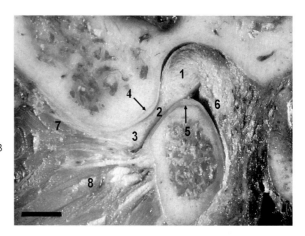

Fig. 4.4 Section through a TM joint: 1, pars posterior; 2, pars intermediate; 3, pars anterior; 4 and 5, fibrocartilage covering the condyle and fossa; 6, inferior lamina of the posterior attachment; 7 and 8, superior and inferior head of the lateral pterygoid muscle. (From Luder with permission.)

the temporal bone. The rotatory movements occur mainly between condyle and disc, while translation occurs between the condyle–disc complex and the temporal fossa (Figs 4.1 and 4.2). Under abnormal conditions, for instance when the disc is displaced from its normal position, translation may also occur between condyle and disc (Fig. 4.3).

Temporal component

The temporal component consists of the concave glenoid fossa and the convex articular tubercle or eminence. Considering the capsular attachments as its boundary, the temporal component of the joint is slightly wider mediolaterally than anteroposteriorly, on average 23 mm and 19 mm respectively. The depth of the fossa and the inclination of the posterior slope of the eminence vary greatly between individuals. Attempts have been made to correlate the inclination of the posterior slope with occlusal characteristics, for instance the inclination of the incisal guidance, but no such correlations have been found.

In the newborn the glenoid fossa is very shallow (almost flat) and develops rapidly during the first years of life; it reaches about half its final shape by the time the eruption of the primary dentition is completed. The rate of development of the eminence reduces at about 5 years of age, and slowly diminishes, stopping by the middle to late teens. This early development of the eminence reflects the changes in the direction of joint loading. This is due to condylar growth, transition from suckling to chewing, and variation in the three-dimensional orientation of the musculature caused by growth of the craniofacial complex.

Posteriorly the fossa is limited by the postglenoid tubercle of the squamous part of the temporal bone and lies just in front of the squamotympanic and petrotympanic fissures.

The articulating part of the temporal component is covered by a thin layer of soft tissue consisting, from the articular surface down to the bone of: (1) a fibrous connective tissue zone; (2) a proliferation zone containing undifferentiated mesenchyme cells (not always present); and (3) a cartilage zone. Its thickness varies anteroposteriorly, being thin in the roof of the fossa and thickest at the articular eminence (Fig. 4.4 – about 0.4 mm at the eminence, 0.2 mm at the slope and 0.05 mm in the fossa). This reflects the fact that the functionally loaded part of the glenoid fossa is not the roof but the eminence, in particular its posterior slope.

Mandibular condyle

The condyle normally has an elliptical shape, and measures on average 20 mm mediolaterally and 10 mm anteroposteriorly. The dimension varies considerably between individuals, with a range of 13–25 mm mediolaterally and 5.5–16 mm anteroposteriorly. The shape of the condyle also presents great interindividual variation.

After the age of 3 years, condylar growth occurs mostly in a mediolateral direction. The anteroposterior dimension does not change significantly, whereas the mediolateral dimension increases by a factor of 2.5 until adulthood.

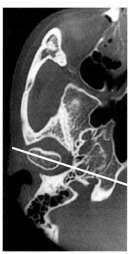 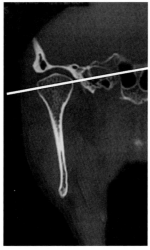

A   B

Fig. 4.5 Computed tomography of the TM joint.
A Horizontal and **B** frontal sections indicate the inclination of the condylar long axis in the horizontal and frontal planes.

Condylar growth stops in females in the late teens but may continue into the twenties in males.

The condyles are not aligned in a transverse axis. On the contrary, their condylar long axes, that is the axis connecting the medial and lateral pole of each condyle, usually converge in a posterosuperior direction, forming an obtuse angle between right and left axes. For imaging purposes, there is a tendency to differentiate between the horizontal and the vertical condylar angle, that is, the angle formed by the condylar axis and the frontal and horizontal planes, respectively. The horizontal condylar angle varies between 0° and 30° with a mean of about 15°, while the vertical condylar angle varies even more (Fig. 4.5).

The condyle is covered by a thin layer of fibrocartilage similar to that of the fossa. The soft tissue layer is thickest superiorly and anteriorly (see Fig. 4.4).

Articular disc

The disc is a fibrocartilaginous structure. In an anteroposterior direction it can be subdivided in three zones: an anterior (foot-like) zone ('pes'), an intermediate (thinner) zone ('pars gracilis') and a posterior (thicker) zone ('pars posterior'). The anterior and posterior zones are also referred to as the anterior and posterior bands (see Fig. 4.4). The posterior band is usually thicker than the anterior band. The disc is composed of densely organised collagen fibres, cartilage-like proteoglycans (CLPGs), elastic fibres and cells that vary from fibrocytes to chondrocytes. The collagen consists mainly of types I

and II. Type II collagen is present especially in areas with CLPGs; which are found mainly in the posterior band. The collagen fibres have a typical pattern distribution: in the intermediate zone the thick collagen bundles are oriented sagittally; anteriorly and posteriorly they enter into the anterior and posterior bands to become interlaced or continuous with the mainly transversally oriented collagen fibres of these disc regions. Other fibres pass through the entire bands to continue into the anterior and posterior disc attachments. The transversely oriented fibres are more pronounced in the posterior band. Thus, in the intermediate part there is a weaker crosslinking of the collagen bundles, making the central part of the disc less resistant to mediolateral shear stresses.

The shape of the disc is well adapted to the form of the condyle and fossa (see Fig. 4.4), and disc shape varies greatly between individuals. For instance, the degree of disc biconcavity depends on the depth of the fossa: in joints with a deep fossa the disc is more concave because the posterior part is thick, while in joints with a shallow fossa the disc is less biconcave, that is, it is more even in thickness. The thickness, and therefore the degree of concavity, also often varies mediolaterally (Fig. 4.6); depending on the shape of the fossa the disc can be thicker medially or laterally.

The disc is avascular and non-innervated, and is flexible in order to:

- adapt its shape to the form of condyle and fossa during mandibular movements
- decrease the stress concentrations due to joint incongruencies and therefore improve load distribution.

This ability depends on disc thickness: the thicker the disc the better its ability to distribute the load. Given that the mechanical properties of the disc facilitate its role as a stress distribution mechanism, it is reasonable to hypothesise that the physical condition of the disc determines the longevity of the joint structures. Therefore, stresses that cause fatigue of the disc might ultimately compromise the primary stress control mechanism of the joint.

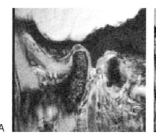 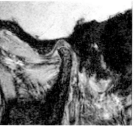

A   B

Fig. 4.6 **A** Lateral and **B** medial magnetic resonance images of a TM joint. The posterior part of the disc can be seen to be thicker medially than laterally.

Joint capsule

Unlike many other joints, the TM joint does not have a circular capsule. A distinct capsule exists only laterally and posteriorly, while medially and anteriorly it is absent or so thin that it can hardly be distinguished from the disc attachments. In these areas, the TM joint wall is formed only by those structures that consist of a superior lamina inserting into the periostium of the temporal bone, and an inferior one inserting into the periostium of the condyle. The lateral joint capsule consists of a prominent inferior disc attachment and a thick capsule.

The capsule is lined with the synovial membrane which continues through a zone of gradual histological transition, i.e. without a distinct boundary, into the fibrous lining of the articular cartilage of condyle, disc and fossa. The similar structure and continuity of the articular and synovial lining tissues suggest that they form a continuous tissue system, the 'articular synovial lining tissue system'. The synovial tissues appear as a folded (areolar) and a smooth (fibrous) membrane. The folded form is at the posterosuperior and anteroinferior attachment, and the smooth form predominates at the anterosuperior and posteroinferior attachment.

The synovial membrane secretes synovial fluid. This is a transudate of extravascular fluid from the capillaries in the intermediate layer of the capsule. As with other synovial joints, it provides nutrition for the cartilage and lubrication, and acts as a heat-dissipating mechanism. With joint motion, some friction inevitably takes place and generates heat. The heat is dissipated by the constant flow of fluid across the synovial membrane into the joint cavity and its subsequent resorption by the subsynovial lymphatics located in the loose areolar tissue between the inner border of synovial cells and the outer fibrous ligaments.

Disc attachments

The attachments that allow the disc to rotate around the condyle and slide anteriorly are particularly important for disc mobility.

Anterior attachments

In this area the superior lamina is thicker than the inferior lamina, especially in the lateral and central areas. It consists of dense collagen fibres that insert into the periostium of the infratemporal surface in front of the eminence. The inferior lamina, which inserts into the condyle more superiorly than the posterior attachment, is composed of loose wavy fibres and forms a small recess of the inferior joint cavity (Figs 4.7 and 4.8). Sparse elastic fibres are found in the inferior lamina.

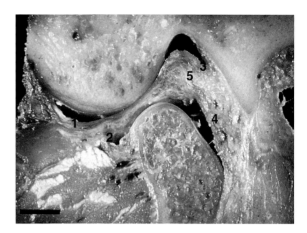

Fig. 4.7 Section through a TM joint. The condyle is in a slightly anterior position. The posterior and anterior attachments and the border between the posterior part of the disc and the bilaminar zone are clearly visible. 1 and 2, superior and inferior laminae of the anterior attachment; 3 and 4, superior and inferior laminae of the posterior attachment; 5, border between posterior band and bilaminar zone. (From Luder with permission.)

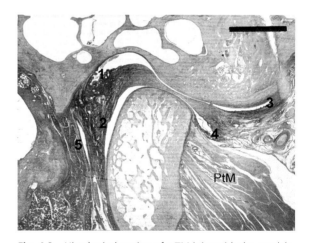

Fig. 4.8 Histological section of a TM joint with the condyle in a slightly anterior position. Note the different disc attachments and the folds in the superior lamina of the posterior attachment. 1, posterosuperior attachment; 2, posteroinferior attachment; 3, anterosuperior attachment; 4, anteroinferior attachment; 5, posterior capsule; PtM, lateral pterygoid muscle. (From Luder 1991 with permission from Schweiser Monatsschrift für Zahnmedizin.)

Lateral and medial attachments

The lateral disc attachment inserts into the lateral pole and contains, in addition to more or less vertically oriented collagen fibres, fibre bundles that are oriented in

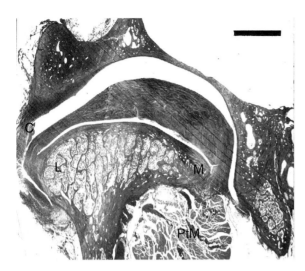

Fig. 4.9 Insertion of the disc to the lateral (L) and medial (M) pole of the condyle. The medial insertion inserts below the pole. A capsule is only visible laterally (C). PtM, lateral pterygoid muscle. (From Luder 1991 with permission from the Schweizer Monatsschrift für Zahnmedizin.)

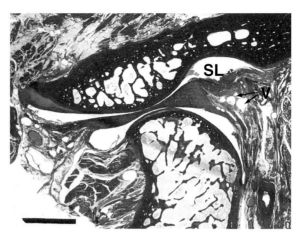

Fig. 4.10 Histological section of a TM joint with the condyle in an anterior position. The superior lamina of the posterior attachment (SL) begins to become stretched, and blood vessels (V) in the retrodiscal pad dilate. This tissue is pulled anteriorly in the retrocondylar space. The opened joint spaces are artefacts. See Fig. 4.11 for comparison in which the posterosuperior lamina is close to the fossa. (From Luder with permission.)

an almost concentric fashion. These fibres insert into the lateral pole from anterior and posterior directions. With an opening rotation of the condyle, posterior fibres are released while the anterior ones are tightened. This allows a firm disc–condyle connection that still permits condylar rotation. The medial capsule consists of a thin superior and a somewhat thicker inferior disc attachment. Unlike the lateral insertion, the medial attachment inserts below the medial pole and is less firm than the lateral attachment (Fig. 4.9).

Posterior attachments

The posterior attachment is normally termed the 'bilaminar zone' or 'retrodiscal pad'. The lower lamina inserts into the periostium of the condyle, the insertion being located more superiorly in the lateral part of the condyle than in the central and medial parts, where it is located approximately 8–10 mm below the vertex of the condyle. The superior lamina inserts into the periostium of the fossa in front of the squamotympanic and petrotympanic fissures. Between these strata lies loose connective tissue with elastic fibres, blood and lymph vessels, nerves and fat tissue. The inferior lamina consists of thick fibres that originate from almost the entire height of the posterior band, and lacks elastic fibres (see Figs 4.7 and 4.8). It can be easily folded during condylar rotation and is inelastic. The superior lamina is thinner than the lower one and also has thinner collagen fibres. The fibres of both laminae

enter the posterior band and become contiguous with the sagittally oriented collagen fibres. Elastic fibres are visible only in the superior lamina and in the posterior capsule. The latter extends from the anterior slope of the post-glenoid tubercle to the condylar neck below the attachment of the lower lamina. This is made up mainly of condensed fibrous tissue.

It has been postulated that the elasticity of the superior lamina should pull back the disc during closing. The content of elastic fibres in the superior lamina is, however, not sufficient to provide this ligament with the elastic force needed to do this. It is more likely that the elastic fibres of the lamina prevent the loose connective tissue from becoming trapped between the articular surfaces during jaw movements. In the closed mouth position the collagen fibres of the superior lamina as well as the synovial lining are extensively folded. During opening or protrusion the superior lamina becomes stretched, allowing the disc to glide anteriorly (Fig. 4.10). Similarly, the anteroinferior lamina becomes stretched during condylar rotation and moves the attachment insertion anteriorly in relation to the disc. Thus, the position of the disc on the moving condyle is controlled by the lateral, and to a lesser extent by the medial as well as by the posteroinferior, disc attachment.

The function of the loose tissue between the two strata and the posterior capsule is to compensate for the changes in pressure that arise when the condyle translates anteriorly. The loose fibroelastic framework allows the

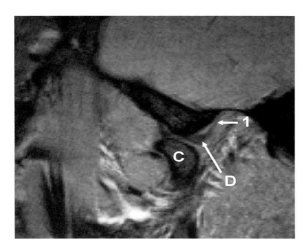

Fig. 4.11 Magnetic resonance image of the condyle–disc complex at maximum mouth opening. The superior lamina of the posterior attachment (1) is located close to the fossa and the disc (D) lies on top of the posterior part of the condyle (C).

blood vessels to expand, producing an enlargement of the volume of this tissue (Fig. 4.10); at full mouth opening there is an increase by a factor between four and five. As a consequence, the posterosuperior lamina is pressed against the fossa and the posteroinferior lamina becomes folded upwards (Fig. 4.11). The expansion of this tissue is due to the dilatation of the venous plexus that is connected medially to the pterygoid plexus located antero-medially to the condyle. On opening, this venous blood can be drawn posteriorly and laterally to fill the enlarged space behind the condyle, and on closing it is pushed out. Pressure compensation is also achieved to a far lesser extent by the inward bulging of the parotid gland and subcutaneous tissue behind the condyle. The bilaminar zone is thus designed to allow rapid volume changes in the retrocondylar space. Lack of a quick pressure compensatory mechanism on opening, closing or translation would prevent smooth condylar movements. Further details may be found in Luder and Bobst (1991) and Scapino (1997).

Disc attachment to muscles

The relationship of the masseter, temporal and in particular of the lateral pterygoid muscles to the TM joint has been the subject of several investigations. There are two forms of disc–muscle attachment:

- Fibrous connections consist of fibrous septa that are perpendicular to the direction of the muscle fibres.

They are continuations of the perimysium that extend into the disc. In the deep masseter and posterior part of the temporal muscle the septa are fine, while at the superior head of the lateral pterygoid muscle the lamellae show an increase in thickness from lateral to medial.

- In muscular insertions, the tendinous end of the muscle fibres insert into the disc. This insertion is present only for the fibres of the superior layer of the superior head of the lateral pterygoid muscle in about 60% of joints. These fibres insert medially into the disc. The remainder of the muscle inserts into the pterygoid fovea above the insertion of the inferior head with fibrous connections. The remaining 40% of the joints, i.e. of the discs, does not have a muscular but only a fibrous connection. When the fibres inserting into the disc are pulled, it is possible to stretch the disc but not to pull it forwards, indicating that an anterior disc displacement cannot be caused by abnormal activity of the superior head. Further details may be found in Meyenberg et al (1986).

Disc position

In maximum intercuspation the posterior band lies above the condyle (see Figs 4.4 and 4.6) and the thin inter-mediate zone is located in front of the condyle between it and the posterior slope of the eminence (see Fig. 4.4). In magnetic resonance images the border between the posterior band and the bilaminar zone is seen to be located superiorly in the majority of cases – in the so-called '12 o'clock' position (see Figs 4.1 and 4.6). Magnetic resonance imaging has also shown that in about one-third of individuals without subjective and objective joint disorders, the posterior band lies anteriorly.

Joint innervation

The TM joint capsule is richly innervated by branches of the trigeminal nerve: the auriculotemporal, masseteric and deep posterior temporal nerves. As with other joints of the body, branches of the nerves innervating the muscles acting upon it also innervate the joint capsule. Small nerve bundles, from the main nerve trunk innervating the joint capsule, also innervate the most peripheral parts of the disc, especially in the anterior and posterior areas. The capsule and retrodiscal pad also contain perivascular nerve fibres.

The trigeminal nerve endings are either:

- free nerve endings that are thought to be nociceptors; or
- mechanoreceptors that are involved in the reflex control of masticatory muscles.

The following receptors have been described: Ruffini endings, Pacinian type endings and Golgi-type endings.

Immunohistochemical staining in the rat TM joint indicated the presence of nerve fibres containing a variety of neuropeptides (neuropeptide Y, vasoactive intestinal peptide, pituitary adenylate cyclase-activating peptide, substance P, calcitonin gene-related peptide) and nitric oxide synthase, in the synovial membrane, the joint capsule and entering the articular disc. Retrograde transport resulted in the appearance of numerous labelled nerve cell bodies in the trigeminal and superior cervical ganglia, and moderate numbers in the nodose, otic, sphenopalatine, stellate and dorsal root ganglia at levels C2–C5. Innervation of the TM joint is therefore complex, and different sensory and autonomic ganglia are involved.

Joint lubrication

The frictional coefficient within a joint is very low, and impairment of joint lubrication has been considered as a possible cause of TM joint disorders. One TM joint disorder considered to be related to impaired joint lubrication is the 'anchored disc' phenomenon that manifests itself by 'closed lock' (Nitzan et al 2002).

The TM joint is subjected to various loading conditions:

- lightly loaded motion with higher speed (for example, during jaw opening/closing or speaking)
- impact loads (for example, during sudden mandibular accelerations, related either to fracture of a hard bolus or trauma)
- fixed steady loads (for example, during sustained clenching).

Under all conditions, lubrication by a viscous fluid layer is essential to protect the articular surfaces. The low friction between the articulating surfaces is most likely to be provided by a combination of boundary and weeping lubrication. Details may be found in Nickel et al (2001) and Nitzan et al (2002). During light loaded motions, the presence of a synovial fluid film due to hydrodynamic effects keeps frictional forces very low. During higher loads at slower gliding speeds of articular surfaces, as well as at the beginning of movement, the main contribution to joint lubrication appears to be fluid squeezed out from the cartilage matrix (weeping lubrication). During extreme loading conditions, ultrafiltration, that is, the motion of fluid into the cartilage matrix, produces a viscous gel that separates and protects the articular surfaces.

CONDYLAR MOVEMENTS

Examples of condylar movements during various types of movement may be found at http://www.dent.unizh.ch/kfs/.

Figure 4.12 shows a lateral view of movement of the condyles during the closing phase of a chewing cycle. The first image represents the position at the beginning of closing. Three features of the closing stroke may be appreciated:

- There is a difference in the velocity of the retrusive movement of both condyles: the ipsilateral or working condyle moves faster posterosuperiorly and reaches its uppermost position in the fossa before the contralateral condyle. In Figure 4.12-4 the working condyle is almost seated in the fossa, while the contralateral condyle is still on the posterior slope. This led to the hypothesis that the ipsilateral condyle acts as a stabilising fulcrum during the so-called 'power stroke', that is, when force is applied to crush food.
- On opening, both condyles translate approximately the same amount and are located just behind the eminence.
- As seen in the compound figure (Fig. 4.12, lower right), the condyle rotates about 10°, far less than during maximum opening (see Fig. 4.1 for comparison). At maximum opening the condyle rotates on average by 30°; during chewing the rotatory component is about 10°. During so small a rotation, only the superior part of the condyle is loaded, and this is the area where the fibrocartilage is thickest.

Rotation versus translation

As already stated, jaw movements occur by a combination of:

- rotation of the condyle against the disc
- translation of the condyle–disc complex.

Both always occur simultaneously during functional movements; that is, opening movements always start with a combination of rotation and translation. However, there is great intra- and interindividual variability in the relationship between condylar rotation and anterior translation during empty opening and closing movements. Three patterns have been described during jaw opening, and four during jaw closing. Opening movements are performed most often (75%) by a constant simultaneous increase in rotation and anterior translation, resulting in a linear relationship between the two components through-out the movement. This means that from the beginning of opening, both condylar rotation and anterior translation of the condyle–disc complex occur together and these two movement components increase constantly throughout the movement. A second pattern (16%) is characterised by marked rotation only at the beginning of opening. The third, less frequently observed, pattern (9%) has a marked initial and final rotatory component.

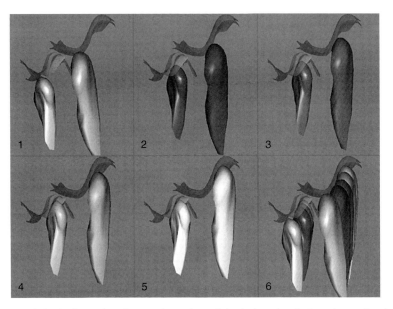

Fig. 4.12 Five positions of the ipsilateral and contralateral condyle during the closing phase of a chewing cycle. The lower right figure is a compound image.

When the data of all recorded movements are considered together, the relationship between rotation and translation in asymptomatic subjects has an almost perfect linear relationship for both opening and closing. On average, condylar rotation increases by approximately 2° per millimetre of anterior translation during opening, and decreases by approximately the same amount of posterior translation during closing (Salaorni & Palla 1994).

The relationship between rotation and translation has clinical implications, and explains the decrease in mouth opening when anterior condylar translation is reduced, as in the case of an anterior disc displacement without reduction. As the degree of mouth opening is mainly determined by the amount of condylar rotation, and a decrease in translation causes a decrease in condylar rotation, it follows that mouth opening must decrease.

Closing movements show a greater variability between rotation and translation (for details, see Salaorni & Palla 1994). The amount of condylar rotation does not differ between males and females, a finding which contrasts with the larger maximum interincisal opening of men compared with women. However, this is not surprising, as the degree of opening measured at the incisors depends not only on the degree of rotation but also on the size of the mandible. Indeed, with the same degree of rotation, the larger the mandible the larger the mouth opening. Consequently, the degree of interincisal opening cannot be considered as a measure of joint mobility or laxity, unless it is corrected for mandibular size.

JOINT LOADING

A question often raised in dentistry is whether or not the TM joint is loaded during function. Computer modelling and recordings in monkeys consistently predict that both joints are loaded during chewing as well as during clenching in eccentric positions. The ipsilateral (working) condyle can be distracted, i.e. unloaded, only when a subject is biting on the third molar, a finding also confirmed with computer simulation and recordings on monkeys. In addition, the measurements of the variation of the minimum condyle–fossa distance in vivo during chewing indicate that both condyles are loaded during the closing phase. As the decrease of the minimum condyle–fossa distance during the closing phase of a chewing stroke is generally larger on the contralateral (non-working) than on the ipsilateral (working) side, there must be a larger compression of the disc on the non-working side. This result is in keeping with the models describing a greater load on the contralateral than on the ipsilateral side during the closing phase of chewing. For detailed results see Palla et al (1997).

JOINT REMODELLING

Joint growth stops at about 18–20 years of age (earlier in men than in women). After that time soft and hard tissues undergo continuous change, i.e. they are continuously remodelled. Articular remodelling is considered as normal adaptation of soft and hard tissues to the load changes within the joint. Progressive and regressive remodelling are described:

- Progressive remodelling is characterized by tissue proliferation, i.e. by an increase in the volume of the remodelled tissue with either higher cell density and/or higher number of cells of a certain phenotype.
- In regressive remodelling there is a decrease in tissue volume and in cell number as well as other signs of tissue degeneration.

Joint remodelling leads to changes in the shape of the condyle and fossa which may disturb normal joint bio-mechanics. This form change may cause a higher degree of incongruency between condyle and fossa so that the disc tissue may undergo greater stress concentration.

Disc remodelling

Biomechanical stimulus is a primary mechanism for signal transduction between chondrocytes and matrix (cell–matrix interactions through integrins) and indirectly between cells and physiological stimuli (cell–molecule interactions through receptors). These signalling pathways are associated with biological regulatory events, such as changes in mechanical loads, which influence these pathways and stimulate remodelling.

In anterior disc displacement, there is:

- an increase in mechanical load in the posterior disc attachment and, depending on the degree of displacement (partial, total, with or without reduction),
- a reduction in compressive load in the intermediate and anterior disc zones.

As a consequence of the posterior band becoming trapped between condyle and fossa, it undergoes fibrotic change:

- The collagen fibres bundles become thicker, more rectilinear, and become oriented parallel to the attach-ment surface. The elastic fibres thin out, vascularity decreases and the fibrotic attachment may appear hyalinised and may contain cells of cartilage phenotype as well as CLPGs.
- In the posterior band, the collagen fibres become aligned in all directions and the transverse bundles may increase in thickness, probably to resist increased tensile stress in the mediolateral direction.
- In the anterior band, rearrangement of the collagen fibres also occurs and, with a decrease in compressive load, the CLPGs disappear. The anterior disc attach-ment to the condyle becomes stretched and the disc may remain stretched or become flexed. In the latter case, collagen fibres on the outside of the flexure are oriented

parallel to the surface, whereas those inside are parallel or transversally oriented.

These changes emphasise the remodelling of a displaced disc to resist functional loads.

OSTEOARTHROSIS

Osteoarthrosis is a degenerative, primarily non-inflammatory joint disease, characterised macroscopically by cartilage degradation and deterioration that may progress to complete cartilage destruction and exposure of subchondral bone. The alteration of the articular surface leads to increased friction during jaw movement and crepitation, which is pathognomonic for this disease. Being primarily non-inflammatory, osteoarthrosis is usually non-painful, or there may be painful episodes that resolve spontaneously. As a result, two forms of osteoarthrosis are described:

- osteoarthrosis without secondary synovitis and no pain
- osteoarthritis with seconday synovitis and pain.

The pathophysiology involves secretion of proteolytic enzymes (metalloproteinases and cathepsin B) by chondrocytes; both cytokine-independent and cytokine-dependent mechanisms are involved (Fig. 4.13):

- *Cytokine-independent mechanism.* This begins as fibrillation of the articular surface, a decrease in the metabolic activity in the most superficial layer and an increase in the water content of the cartilage. As a con-sequence, chondrocytes do not receive oxygen and nutrients by slow diffusion from synovial fluid through the cartilage but directly, so that their metabolic activity changes from anaerobic to aerobic.

  This causes a phenotypic alteration of the chondrocytes that dedifferentiate to form cells that have the charac-teristics of both fibroblasts (fibroblastic metaplasia) and hypertrophic chondrocytes (phenotypic modulation). The dedifferentiated chondrocytes synthesise matrix components that are typical for fibroblasts: collagen type I, III and X, and proteoglycans with a higher molecular mass.

  They also proliferate and secrete cathepsin B, an aggressive enzyme that leads to degradation of all cartilage components. This enzyme is also capable of inactivating the tissue inhibitors of the matrix metallo-proteinases (TIMP-1 and TIMP-2), which are also proteolytc enzymes. TIMP-1 and TIMP-2 also inhibit blood vessel formation in the cartilage.

- *Cytokine-dependent mechanism.* Chondrocytes usually secrete proteolytic enzymes in a non-harmful concentration controlled by extracellular inhibitors. In osteoarthrosis the production of proteolytic enzymes increases. Synovial

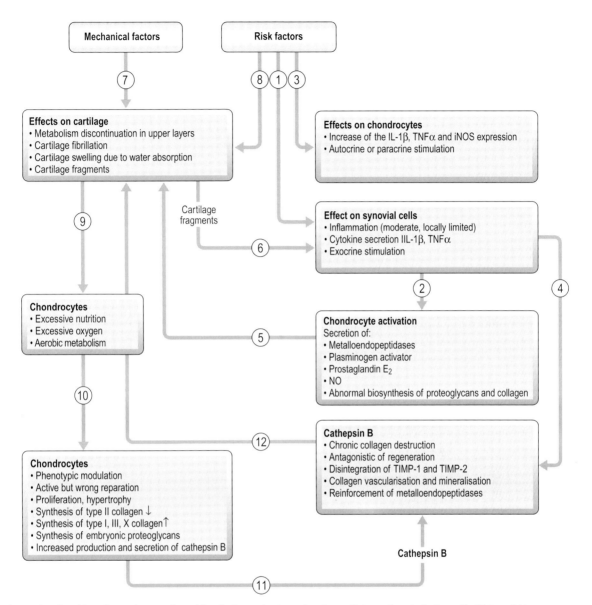

Fig. 4.13 Cytokine-dependent and cytokine-independent mechanisms. Osteoarthrosis (osteoarthritis) could be determined by the cascade of the events 3, 4, 5, 9, 10, 11, 12, with the sequence 9, 10, 11, 12 and the mechanical factors 7 determining the chronicity of the osteoarthrotic process (From Baici, with permission from RC Libri, Milano.)

cells are stimulated to secrete cytokines (interleukin (IL-1β) and tumour necrosis factor alpha (TNFα)), which diffuse into the fibrocartilage and stimulate condrocytes to produce metalloproteinases. These proteolytic enzymes degrade the collagen matrix, as with cathepsin B.

Further destructive effects of cytokines involve suppression of collagen types II and IX, the inhibition of proteoglycan synthesis and stimulation of prostaglandin E_2 synthesis. The free cartilage fragments

produced by cartilage degeneration may stimulate synovial cells to further secrete cytokines, producing a vicious circle. This cytokine-induced mechanism results in local painful inflammation with prostaglandin E_2 secretion.

These cytokine-dependent and cytokine-independent mechanisms may coexist (Fig. 4.13). It is likely that the cytokine-independent mechanism plays a central role in chronic, non-painful phases of the disease, while the cytokine-dependent mechanism dominates during painful episodes. The final stages of osteoarthrosis are dominated by cartilage that is unable to resist functional load. The weakened cartilage loses its biomechanical function, becomes atrophic and the chondrocytes die by apoptosis. As a consequence of vascularisation, osteophytes form and may disturb joint biomechanics.

Histological studies indicate that TM joint osteoarthrosis has a similar pathophysiological mechanism as joints with hyaline cartilage:

- The first signs are chondrocyte proliferation and an increase in their metabolic activity. This reparative process allows osteoarthrosis to remain asymptomatic for several years.
- Later, cartilage volume increases due to an increase in water content and the surface becomes irregular. Chondrocytes produce proteolytic enzymes that lead to a disintegration of the collagen matrix. The surface develops deep fissures and loss of cartilage due to intra-articular frictional forces. Islands of chondrocytes become visible near the deep fissures.
- In the final phase these become larger. As a consequence of the proteolytic destruction of collagen fibres and of proteoglycans, fibrocartilage disappears, chondrocytes die and the subchondral bone becomes exposed.

There are endogenous (age, gender, genetic disposition and race) and exogenous (joint form and instability, traumatic lesions and overloading) risk factors. The osteoarthrotic process does not necessarily progress to complete degeneration of fibrocartilage. It is likely that mechanical factors determine the progression of the disease. Thus, all therapies that decrease TM joint loading (e.g. avoiding parafunction) are important in decreasing the risk of progression.

Acknowledgement

The author thanks Dr H.U. Luder for providing Figures 4.4, 4.7–4.10.

References

Luder H U, Bobst P 1991 Wall architecture and disc attachment of the human temporomandibular joint. Schweizer Monatsschrift für Zahnmedizin 101: 557–570

Meyenberg K, Kubik S, Palla S 1986 Relationships of the muscles of mastication to the articular disc of the temporomandibular joint. Schweizer Monatsschrift für Zahnmedizin 96: 815–834

Nickel J C, Iwasaki L R, Feely D E et al 2001 The effect of disc thickness and trauma on disc surface friction in the porcine temporomandibular joint. Archives of Oral Biology 46: 155–162

Nitzan D W, Goldfarb A, Gati I et al 2002 Changes in the reducing power of synovial fluid from temporomandibular joints with 'anchored disc phenomenon'. Journal of Oral Maxillofacial Surgery 60: 735–740

Palla S, Krebs M, Gallo L M 1997 Jaw tracking and temporomandibular joint animation. In: McNeill C (ed) Science and practice of occlusion. Quintessence Chicago, pp 365–378

Salaorni C, Palla S 1994 Condylar rotation and anterior translation in healthy human temporomandibular joints. Schweizer Monatsschrift für Zahnmedizin 104: 415–422

Scapino R P 1997 Morphology and mechanism of the jaw joint. In: McNeill C (ed) Science and practice of occlusion. Quintessence Chicago, pp 23–40

Further reading

Baici A, Lang A, Zwicky R, Müntener K 2003 Cathepsin B in osteoarthritis: uncontrolled proteolysis at the wrong place. Seminars in Arthritis and Rheumatism (in press)

Bibb C A, Pullinger A G, Baldioceda F 1992 The relationship of undifferentiated mesenchymal cells to TMJ articular tissue thickness [published erratum appears in Journal of Dental Research 72:88]. Journal of Dental Research 71: 1816–1821

Gallo L M, Nickel J C, Iwasaki L R, Palla S 2000 Stress-field translation in the healthy human temporomandibular joint. Journal of Dental Research 79: 1740–1746

Hannam A G 1994 Musculoskeletal biomechanics in the human jaw. In: Zarb G A, Carlsson G E, Sessle B J et al (eds) Temporomandibular joint and masticatory muscle disorders. 2nd edn. Munksgaard Copenhagen; pp 101–127

Luder H U 1993 Articular degeneration and remodeling in human temporomandibular joints with normal and abnormal disc position. Journal of Orofacial Pain 7: 391–402

Morani V, Previgliano V, Schierano G M et al 1994 Innervation of the human temporomandibular joint capsule and disc as revealed by immunohistochemistry for neurospecific markers. Journal of Orofacial Pain 8: 36–41

Nickel J C, McLachlan K R 1994 In vitro measurement of the frictional properties of the temporomandibular joint disc. Archives of Oral Biology 39: 323–331

Nickel J C, Iwasaki L R, McLachlan K R 1997 Effect of the physical environment on growth of the temporomandibular joint. In: McNeill C (ed) Science and practice of occlusion. Quintessence Chicago, pp 115–124

Scapino R P, Mills D K 1997 Disc displacement internal derangements In: McNeill C (ed) Science and practice of occlusion. Quintessence Chicago, pp 220–234

Uddman R, Grunditz T, Kato J et al 1998 Distribution and origin of nerve fibers in the rat temporomandibular joint capsule. Anatomy and Embryology (Berlin) 197: 273–282

Wilkinson T M, Crowley C M 1994 A histologic study of retrodiscal tissues of the human temporomandibular joint in the open and closed position. Journal of Orofacial Pain 8: 7–17

ASSESSMENT OF THE OCCLUSION

5 Clinical occlusal analysis

I. Klineberg

Synopsis

The assessment of the teeth is an integral part of treatment planning in restorative dentistry. A broad distribution of tooth contacts disperses vectors of force from function and parafunction over many teeth and avoids force concentration on a limited number of teeth.

Clinical occlusal analysis allows a detailed assessment of tooth contacts in retruded contact position (RCP), median occlusal position (MOP) and lateral and protrusive jaw excursions. Modification of tooth contacts in these jaw positions may be indicated in restorative care. Occlusal adjustment and selective grinding are discussed in Chapter 14.

Indications of parafunctional tooth wear are described and the value of provocation tests linked with bruxofacets is discussed. Provocation tests may indicate an association between the particular tooth wear pattern with jaw posture and orofacial symptoms. This information may be of special importance in restorative treatment planning.

Key points

- Jaw guidance techniques are described
- Tooth contacts in MOP and RCP are identified with ultrafine plastic tapes, and their relevance is described
- Lateral guidance, balancing contacts or interferences, and mediotrusive contacts or interferences are specified
- Bruxofacets are identified as evidence of parafunction, and whether there is a combination of attrition and erosion

- Provocation tests are described to determine whether they evoke clinical symptoms:
  - temporomandibular joint provocation test to determine the presence of TM joint pain or discomfort with clenching on a unilateral posterior support; and
  - jaw muscle provocation test to determine the effect on jaw muscles of clenching in intercuspal position (ICP) ('centric bruxing') and clenching with opposing bruxofacets in contact

INTRODUCTION

In the context of occlusion representing both static and dynamic tooth relationships and the integrated action of the jaw muscles and TM joints (see Ch. 1), a comprehensive assessment of the occlusion includes:

- assessment of the positional relationships of the teeth and interarch tooth contacts in 'centric' and eccentric jaw positions
- jaw mobility measurement to determine TM joint function
- jaw muscle palpation following a defined protocol.

The Research Diagnostic Criteria for Temporomandibular Disorders (RDC/TMD) of Dworkin and LeResche (1992) are recognised as the international benchmark for TMD assessment (Truelove et al 1992). This specific clinical procedure has been accepted as a standard TMD assessment and follows studies on validation of data collection by clinicians calibrated against a gold standard. This development is an important step in standardising clinical assessment to justify comparison of clinical studies.

One of the shortcomings of studies on TMD assessment and management has been the lack of a standardised approach to experimental design and clinical assessment (Antczak-Bouckoms 1995). This has prevented valid data

Table 5.1 Tooth contact identification

- **MOP contacts** are marked with red tape to identify functional contacts as distinct from RCP contacts (Fig. 5.2D, E).
- **RCP contacts** are marked with black tape following gentle operator jaw guidance (Fig. 5.2A, B) and the distribution of contacts compared with MOP contacts. Optimum jaw support in RCP suggests bilateral simultaneous contacts on some, or ideally all, posterior teeth. Often only unilateral contacts are present in RCP.
- **A slide from RCP to ICP** may be examined (black tape) by having the patient bite after the initial contact in RCP. This will bring the jaw into ICP and a slide from RCP to ICP, if present, will be observed by the movement of the lower incisor teeth. The slide may have anterior, lateral and/or vertical components; and will be distinctly marked by the black tape.
- **Lateral guidance** is marked with green tape to be distinct from MOP and RCP contacts, to show which teeth (anterior and/or posterior) provide guidance. If anterior guidance is on the canine teeth, whether the tape marks are on the mesial or distal area of the lingual surface is noted (Fig. 5.2G–J).

comparison. It is hoped that the standardised and validated RDC/TMD protocol will encourage multicentre studies and, as a result, the development of large databases for analysis.

This chapter will discuss the details of an assessment of jaw and tooth relationships and will not include the assessment of the TM joints and jaw muscles. These topics are comprehensively described in Chapters 7 and 8, respectively.

A detailed assessment of the static and dynamic relationships of teeth is important in clinical assessment for all aspects of dental practice. The information obtained will provide an understanding of the specific tooth relationships associated with function and parafunction, upon which treatment will be based. The number of tooth contacts around the arch relates directly to jaw muscle activity (Ferrario et al 2002). This is important for prognosis and management of treatment provided, and allows the clinician to more confidently manage the wishes and expectations of patients. It is recognised that, in the older patient, loss of posterior teeth may nevertheless allow appropriate jaw function (Witter et al 2001).

CLINICAL OCCLUSAL ASSESSMENT

Clinical assessment of tooth contact details requires operator confidence in determining jaw positions with guidance, and the use of high-quality ultrafine marking tapes (for example, GHM Foil, Gebr. Hansel-Medizinal, Nurtingen, Germany; Ivoclar/Vivadent, Schaan, Liechtenstein) to accurately determine tooth contact and jaw relationships. These ultrafine tapes minimise contact artefacts and clearly indicate tooth contact details. It is recognised that operator experience is important in consistency of tooth contact markings and that a gold standard approach has not been defined (Millstein & Maya 2001, Harper & Setchell 2002).

Table 5.2 Clinical occlusal assessment requirements

- GHM Foil × 3 (black, red, green) to mark teeth in a specific sequence
- Miller holders × 2 to support GHM Foil for bilateral assessment
- Gauze to dry teeth to allow the ultrafine tape to mark the teeth
- Patient is seated in a dental chair with appropriate lighting
- Assessment is ideally carried out with patient lying supine; alternatively it is possible for patients to be seated upright
- A dental assistant is helpful for supporting the Miller holders

A practical approach in clinical assessment is the use of different coloured plastic tapes (GHM Foils) for identifying specific tooth contacts. For convenience, red, black and green tapes are recommended to allow comparisons to be made, as described in Table 5.1. (See Chapter 1 for revision of jaw and tooth positions.)

Table 5.2 lists the requirements for clinical occlusal assessment.

Retruded contact position

Jaw guidance into RCP may be carried out using chin, chin and jaw, or bilateral jaw guidance. Each clinical approach is satisfactory, but requires practice and experience to gain confidence in the ability to guide the jaw reproducibly. The confidence of the clinician is often challenged by the difficulty that most patients have in relaxing the jaw to allow guidance into RCP (Figs 5.1 and Fig. 5.2A–D).

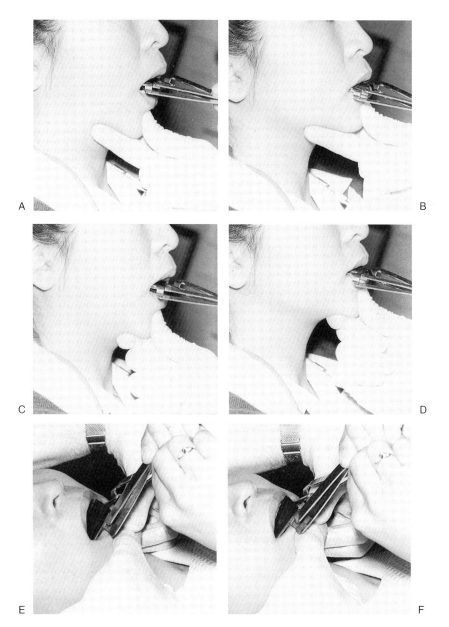

A

B

C

D

E

F

Fig. 5.1 Jaw guidance techniques. **A, B** Jaw guidance obtained by supporting the chin point with the thumb and the lower border of the jaw bilaterally with the index finger and middle finger. The jaw is rotated open and closed with the axis of rotation at the condyles. The assistant supports the Miller holders and recording tape. **C, D** Jaw guidance obtained by supporting the chin point with the thumb and index finger. The same procedure as above is followed in obtaining centric relation tooth contacts. The assistant supports the Miller holders and recording tape. **E, F** Bilateral jaw guidance with the patient lying supine. The jaw is guided with each thumb depressing the chin while the fingertips support the lower border of the jaw. The head is stabilised by the operator seated at the 10 or 11 o'clock position with the head between the chest and inner surface of the left arm (for a right-handed operator). Firm bilateral support, with gentle guidance and the presence of the sensitive fingerpads along the lower border of the jaw, provides an excellent means of accurately recording and testing retruded jaw position or centric relation contacts in the dentate patient. (From Klineberg 1991, with permission.)

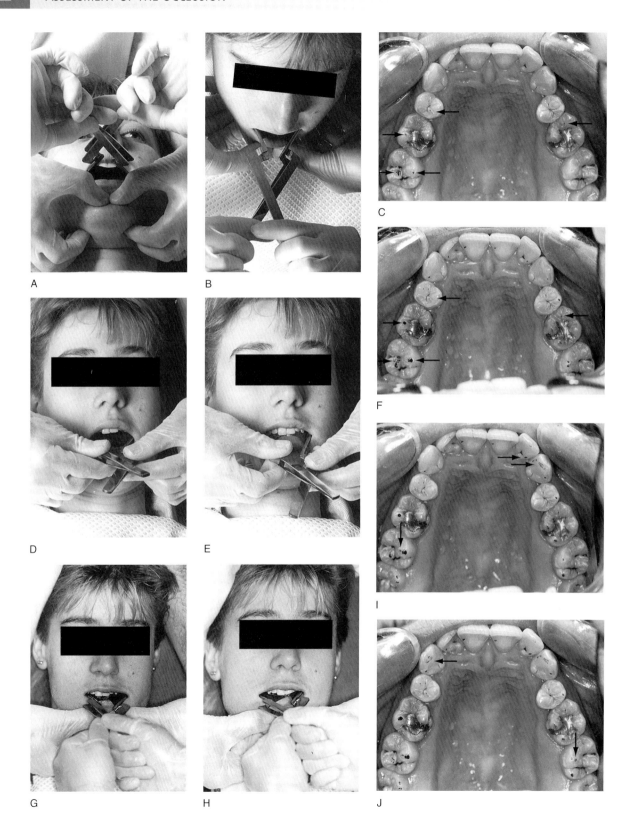

A

B

C

D

E

F

G

H

I

J

Fig. 5.2   Clinical recording of jaw positions. **A, B** Clinical recording of retruded jaw position (RP) with bilateral manual jaw guidance by the clinician. The dental assistant is supporting Miller holders for right and left quadrant recordings with black foil. **C** RP contacts marked with tape (arrows). Definite unilateral tooth contacts are seen on teeth 1.6 (lingual incline of distobuccal cusp), 1.7 (heaviest contact on distobuccal cusp, also on mesiolingual cusp), lighter contact on 1.4 (buccal incline of lingual cusp) and 2.6 (anterior fossa). **D, E** Clinical recording of MOP. The clinician holds Miller holders for right and left quadrant recordings with red foil. MOP contact is obtained by the patient snapping the teeth together (**E**) sharply from a jaw opened position (**D**). The tape marks provide a pattern of functional tooth contacts. **F** MOP contacts are seen to be distributed around the arch in comparison with RP contacts in **C**. Definite supporting contacts are seen on the right: 1.1 (mesial and distal – darker); 1.2 (distal); 1.3 (distal); 1.4 (lingual incline of buccal cusp – light); 1.6 (lingual incline of distobuccal cusp – dark, and lingual groove on amalgam); and 1.7 (mesiolingual cusp tip – dark, and lingual incline of distobuccal cusp posterior to the RP contact). Contacts on the left: 2.1 (mesial); 2.2 (distal); 2.3 (distal); 2.4 (distobuccal cusp incline); 2.6 (mesiolingual and distolingual cusp tips); and 2.7 (mesiolingual and distolingual cusp tips). Original RP contacts are arrowed to indicate clearly the differences between RP and MOP. **G** Lateral jaw guidance to the left. **H** Lateral jaw guidance to the right. **I** Lateral guidance to the left provided by tooth contacts (arrowed) on 2.3 (mesial – major guidance), 2.2 (distolingual) and 1.7 (buccal incline of mesiolingual cusp). **J** Lateral guidance to the right provided by tooth contacts (arrowed) on 1.3 (mesiolingual) and 2.7 (buccal incline of mesiolingual cusp). (From Klineberg 1991, with permission.)

Median occlusal position

Median occlusal position is examined with a different coloured tape (red) to assess the distribution of functional contacts and whether this contact distribution is different from RCP. The optimum tooth arrangement provides multiple bilateral simultaneous contacts, often on all posterior teeth, and, if the anterior tooth arrangement allows (depending on degree of overjet), there may be lighter anterior tooth contacts as well (Fig. 5.2 D–F).

Lateral tooth guidance

The physical features of tooth guidance vary with the intraarch tooth arrangement and the interarch relationships of anterior and posterior teeth, and are described in Chapter 1.

Lateral guidance from RCP (gentle operator guidance only) is examined with tape (green) and the presence of mediotrusive and/or laterotrusive contacts or interferences will be identified by tape marks on the teeth concerned (Fig. 5.2 G–J).

PARAFUNCTIONAL TOOTH WEAR

Parafunctional jaw movements are those movements of the jaw not related to function, that is, not related to mastication, swallowing and speech, facial expression, etc., and jaw postures both with and without tooth contact.

The most common presenting form of tooth contact parafunction from clinical observation appears to be lateroprotrusive parafunction. This may be destructive to teeth and to articular tissues. It may in some instances lead to muscle fatigue and myogenic pain. Sustained jaw

muscle contraction has been shown in clinical studies of healthy adults to evoke a dull ache in the face, temple or forehead, similar to the pain described by patients (Clark et al 1984). In addition, clenching in an eccentric jaw position, that is, not at ICP (centric occlusion, CO), is likely to more readily lead to jaw muscle pain and tenderness to palpation. In eccentric lateroprotrusive or protrusive jaw positions, the jaw muscle system has less resistance to loading, especially when there are no posterior supporting tooth contacts on laterotrusive (working) and mediotrusive (non-working) sides. In centric bruxism posterior tooth support best resists loading, yet muscle pain has been described with centric clenching (see Wänman 1995, for review). Table 5.3 summarises tooth contacts and non-tooth contact parafunction.

An occlusal analysis form allows standardised documentation of tooth contact details for restorative treatment planning (Fig. 5.3). Tooth contacts are indicated by circling the appropriate teeth of the odontograms.

- ICP/MOP. For clinical occlusal analysis MOP is recorded (red tape), followed by RCP contacts (black tape).
- A slide from RCP to ICP (in 90% of individuals) is identified (black tape) by asking the patient to bite on the teeth once the initial RCP contact is determined by clinician guidance. The black tape mark is usually distinct, and the presence of a slide may also be observed through the movement of the lower incisor teeth with biting from initial RCP contact as the jaw slides into ICP. The slide dimensions may also be listed on the form.
- Laterotrusive contacts are identified (green tape), with operator guidance, as the patient moves the jaw from RCP into right and then left laterotrusion. Initial lateral guidance is also indicated on the form.

Table 5.3 Parafunction

Tooth contact parafunction includes:
• Jaw clenching (centric bruxism)
• Jaw grinding (bruxism), which occurs in a lateroprotrusive direction
• Tapping of teeth
• Forced postures of the jaw in which teeth may also be inlocked (such as holding the jaw forward in protrusion with the anterior teeth inlocked in a class II relationship), or in a lateroprotrusive position

Non-tooth contact jaw postures include:
• Holding the jaw in a fixed posture without tooth contact, usually with a varying degree of protrusion; which may be a deliberate attempt to improve facial aesthetics
• Pipe smoking
• Nail biting, pencil biting
• Thumb or finger sucking, particularly in children

• Protrusive contacts from RCP to edge-to-edge contacts are identified (green tape).

• Bruxofacets are observed with the use of a dental mirror and light reflection from tooth surfaces which show signs of wear; these surfaces are usually highly reflective with a good light source. Tooth surface loss is graded (see code at base of table) for both attrition and erosion.

• Vertical dimension is determined in the customary way by observing lower face height proportion and facial aesthetics.

Once the occlusal features are listed, the details may be scored by adding the number of tooth contacts, the RCP–ICP slide dimensions, and the score for tooth surface loss.

Score values are an indication of the degree of tooth contact and surface loss and may be used for comparison for case maintenance in the longterm, or for comparison between patients.

Parafunction may occur during the day (diurnal parafunction) or may also occur at night (nocturnal parafunction or sleep bruxism). It is common for people to be unaware of either diurnal or nocturnal parafunction. However, many patients presenting for treatment with signs and symptoms of parafunction are aware of their daytime habit. Night bruxism is often drawn to the attention of the offender by their room-mate or sleeping partner, and parents often observe this habit in children.

Bruxism may occur at any age and is often noticed in children by their parents. Bruxism in children has been reported to have a similar aetiology to that occurring in adults. Clinical studies provide strong evidence that parafunction, and bruxism especially, are not caused by local dental factors, that is, there is no association between tooth arrangement or tooth contact interferences (from RCP to ICP, mediotrusive or balancing interferences) and the aetiology of parafunction (Seligman et al 1988). There is now strong evidence to indicate that parafunction, especially sleep bruxism, is induced within the central nervous system and is recognised as a sleep disorder (Lavigne et al 1999, Bader & Lavigne 2000, Lobbezoo & Naeije 2001).

Clinical signs

Clinical signs are summarised in Table 5.4. The most common presenting sign is wear on teeth, and attritional wear often presents in conjunction with erosion and abrasion (Bartlett et al 1998, Young 2002). The rate of tooth surface loss is usually of the order of 50 μm per year for posterior teeth (Seligman & Pullinger 1995), and there is a non-linear relationship with age. It was shown by Seligman and Pullinger (1995) that the degree of attrition does not continue to increase in a linear manner with age, and that canine or laterotrusive attrition occurs to a greater degree and more rapidly than posterior attrition. The laterotrusive component of parafunction initially provides some protection of posterior tooth wear. Once reduced anterior guidance develops, the rate of attritional wear increases. However, the presence of wear facets (bruxofacets) are clear evidence of parafunction. It has been determined that approximately 75–80% of tooth surface loss (attrition) can be attributed to parafunction and the remainder to function (which may include erosion) (Seligman & Pullinger 1995). The facets can usually be matched between opposing tooth surfaces. Figure 5.4 shows bruxofacets of varying severity.

During bruxing (particularly sleep bruxism) and centric clenching, the customary controls of jaw movement appear to be absent and tooth contact duration may be sustained. Isometric jaw muscle contraction occurs with increased motor unit contributions, together with the generation of bite forces which may be greater than those occurring during mastication and swallowing. Sustained and repeated tooth contact results in the development of bruxofacets with progressive loss of tooth structure.

The loss of permanent tooth structure occurring on contact surfaces of opposing teeth is usually clearly evident in adults, and early signs of tooth wear may also be seen in teenagers and young adults as the cardinal sign of a parafunctional habit. Since parafunctional clenching and grinding usually occur with the jaw eccentrically placed, bruxofacets are readily seen on the contact surfaces of the teeth providing lateral guidance (usually the incisor and canine teeth). The loss of tooth structure varies widely in different individuals and is a function of several variables including:

OCCLUSAL ANALYSIS

JAW RELATIONSHIP: ant-post:............................... vertical:............................transverse:........................

(Angle molar relationship) (incisor relationship) (crossbite)

ICP/MOP (red)

```
        1 │ 2
8 7 6 5 4 3 2 1 │ 1 2 3 4 5 6 7 8
8 7 6 5 4 3 2 1 │ 1 2 3 4 5 6 7 8
        4 │ 3
```

No. of contracts ☐

LATEROTRUSION R (green)

```
        1 │ 2
8 7 6 5 4 3 2 1 │ 1 2 3 4 5 6 7 8

8 7 6 5 4 3 2 1 │ 1 2 3 4 5 6 7 8
        4 │ 3
```

No. of contracts ☐

PROTRUSION (green)

```
        1 │ 2
8 7 6 5 4 3 2 1 │ 1 2 3 4 5 6 7 8

8 7 6 5 4 3 2 1 │ 1 2 3 4 5 6 7 8
        4 │ 3
```

No. of contracts ☐

RCP (black)

```
        1 │ 2
8 7 6 5 4 3 2 1 │ 1 2 3 4 5 6 7 8
8 7 6 5 4 3 2 1 │ 1 2 3 4 5 6 7 8
        4 │ 3
```

No. ☐

LATEROTRUSION L (green)

```
        1 │ 2
8 7 6 5 4 3 2 1 │ 1 2 3 4 5 6 7 8

8 7 6 5 4 3 2 1 │ 1 2 3 4 5 6 7 8
        4 │ 3
```

No. ☐

BRUXOFACETS

```
        1 │ 2
8 7 6 5 4 3 2 1 │ 1 2 3 4 5 6 7 8

8 7 6 5 4 3 2 1 │ 1 2 3 4 5 6 7 8
        4 │ 3
```

No. ☐

SLIDE (black)

RCP – ICP distance ant-post .... mm

vertical .... mm

lateral displacement .... mm

R or L

INITIAL LATERAL GUIDANCE: R L

(tick box) maxillary tooth ☐ ☐

mesial ☐ ☐

distal ☐ ☐

TOOTH SURFACE

	Inc	can	prem	mol
Attrition*	☐	☐	☐	☐
Erosion*	☐	☐	☐	☐

VERTICAL DIMENSION:

(tick box)

optimal	reduced	severely reduced	open bite anterior	lateral
☐	☐	☐	☐	☐

Scoring the form:

No. of contracts RCP........ Lat. R ...... Lat. L .... Pro .... Score ☐

Slide: **Ant-Post:** 0; 0 –1.0; 1.0 –1.5; 1.5 –2; **Vert:** 0; 0 –1.0; 1.0 –1.5; 1.5 –2;**Lat:** 0; 0 –1.0; 1.0 –1.5; 1.5 –2; Score ☐

    Score 0 1   2   3   0 1 2   3   0 1   2   3

Tooth surface loss

Bruxofacets: No. of teeth with attrition.............. attrition guide**.................. Score ☐

Total ☐

Erosion: erosion.............. erosion guide**.................. Score ☐

**Tooth surface loss guide :

0 – nil; 1 – only enamel; 2 – dentine; 3 – dentine extensively; 4 – dentine and secondary dentine;

Fig. 5.3 Occlusal analysis form. Clinical occlusal analysis may be standardised by completing an occlusal analysis form.

Table 5.4 Parafunction: clinical signs

Teeth
- Wear on teeth and restorations; degree of wear on teeth depends on:
  - enamel hardness
  - interocclusal forces generated and their duration
  - frequency of habit
- Mobility and spreading of teeth
- Fractured cusps and split teeth

Muscles
- Muscle fatigue and/or pain
- Muscle hypertrophy, especially masseter
- Elevated masseter EMG

TM joints
- Possible overloading
- Articular sounds (popping, clicking)
- Internal derangement
  - reciprocal click
  - closed-lock
- Radiographic changes in condyle contour

- duration of tooth contact during each episode
- frequency of parafunctional episodes
- bite force developed during the habit
- whether there is static clenching or dynamic grinding of tooth surfaces
- abrasion resistance of enamel.

Functional jaw movements of chewing, swallowing and speech comprise a relatively small proportion of tooth contact duration. However, in addition, parafunctional clenching occurs in most, if not all, individuals. It may be diurnal during periods of concentration, and nocturnal during sleep, and may be provoked by emotional stress, either experienced or anticipated, or as a component of a sleep disorder. Each of these triggers is associated with a change in central nervous system drive to jaw muscle motoneurones, which leads to an increase in:

- tooth contact time
- muscle contraction force and duration, and
- may also lead to increased loading of articular tissues in tension or compression.

PROVOCATION TESTS

Provocation tests are a useful component of occlusal assessment. They are used to provoke a response in the jaw muscles or TM joints, or both, that may match symptoms or concerns that a patient has been experiencing and may or may not have reported.

Jaw mobility as part of TM joint assessment could be regarded as a provocation test. However, those described in this chapter are associated with bite force for assessment of the teeth, the TM joints and the jaw muscles.

TM joint provocation test

- The patient is asked to bite on a posterior support (for example, cotton roll or wooden spatula – 2 mm thick) placed in the first molar region, separately one side at a time, for 30 seconds.
- Pain or discomfort may be experienced in the contralateral joint or joint area from the effects of compression or tension loading of the joint.
- This occurs as the jaw rotates around the ipsilateral posterior support acting as a fulcrum. Symptoms of discomfort may be linked with the patient's concerns and assist in diagnosis and management.
- On the other hand, the test may not evoke any symptoms or sensation.

Jaw muscle provocation test

- The patient is asked to bite in ICP (CO) – so-called 'centric clenching' for 30 seconds.
  - Pain, discomfort, muscle fatigue (weakness or tiredness) may be provoked and may be similar to symptoms that the patient has experienced in the head, face and/or jaws. This suggests that a parafunctional clenching habit may be the cause of such symptoms.
  - On the other hand, this test may not evoke any symptoms.
- Where there is evidence of parafunctional tooth wear, clenching on the bruxofacets for 30 seconds will reproduce the parafunctional habit.
  - Bruxofacets on anterior teeth can usually be matched with the jaw in a protrusive or lateroprotrusive position.
  - The patient is often unaware of this jaw posture habit, and may be very surprised at the forced and often uncomfortable nature of the jaw position.
  - The matching of the bruxofacets in these jaw positions should be carefully explained to the patient: the use of a face mirror is helpful to visually explain the jaw postures that have unconsciously developed.
  - A careful explanation of the parafunctional habit, emphasising that these specific jaw positions which cause the wear patterns on the teeth are not associated with chewing, swallowing or talking, is an important step in patient education.
  - This is a key feature in the conservative management of parafunctional clenching and its many effects.

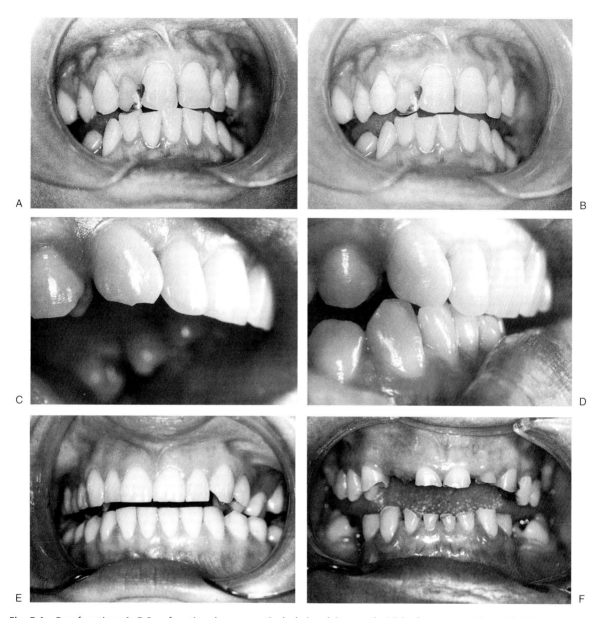

Fig. 5.4 Parafunction. **A, B** Parafunctional wear particularly involving tooth 4.2 is also apparent in tooth 1.1. A marked overbite and overjet required lateroprotrusive jaw posturing for these tooth contacts to occur. Parafunction was present before the inlay was fitted in tooth 1.2, but the presence of the inlay has caused accelerated wear on tooth 4.2. **C, D** Parafunctional wear in its earliest stages involving tooth 1.3 most clearly. Such wear is unrelated to function, and the eccentric posturing of the jaw to gain tooth contact causes physical loading on teeth, TM joints and muscles. The signs on the teeth are obvious; however, deterioration in TM joints and muscles is not obvious and continues until pain or dysfunction occurs, and the patient then presents for treatment. The patient was an 18-year-old student. **E** Parafunctional wear indicated by flattening of incisal edges of incisor teeth at a more advanced stage than in **A–D**. The patient was a 23-year-old dental student and a single parent. **F** Parafunctional wear of an advanced nature in a 43-year-old male showing marked destruction of tooth structure. Such wear is unrelated to functional tooth contacts. There are also components of erosion and abrasion. The wear on anterior teeth has been accelerated by collapse of posterior segments with tooth loss (3.5, 3.6 and 4.5, 4.6) and tilting and drifting of teeth adjacent to the spaces.

The focus on patient education is an important component of the management of patient needs. The use of a tailored self-care programme for TMD has been assessed in a randomised controlled trial by Dworkin et al (2002) and shown to be equally as effective as other treatments in managing TMD. The data indicated that there was reduced TMD pain, reduced jaw muscle tenderness, and an enhanced ability to cope with any residual TMD.

References

Antczak-Bouckoms A A 1995 Epidemiology of research for temporomandibular disorders. Journal of Orofacial Pain 9:226–234

Bader G, Lavigne G 2000 Sleep bruxism; an overview of an oro-mandibular sleep movement disorder. Sleep Medicine Review 4:27–43

Bartlett D W, Coward P Y, Nikkah C, Wilson R F 1998 The prevalence of tooth wear in a cluster sample of adolescent school children and its relationship with potential explanatory factors. British Dental Journal 184:125–129

Clark G T, Beemsterboer P L, Jacobson R 1984 The effect of sustained sub-maximal clenching on maximum biteforce in myofascial pain dysfunction patients. Journal of Oral Rehabilitation 11:387–391

Dworkin S F, LeResche L 1992 Research diagnostic criteria for temporomandibular disorders: review, criteria, examinations and specifications, critique. Journal of Craniomandibular Disorders: Facial and Oral Pain 6:301–355

Dworkin S F, Huggins K H, Wilson L et al 2002 A randomised clinical trial using research diagnostic criteria for temporomandibular disorders – Axis II to target clinical cases for a tailored self-care TMD treatment program. Journal of Orofacial Pain 16:48–63

Ferrario V F, Serrao G, Dellavia C, Caruso E, Sforza C 2002 Relationship between number of occlusal contacts and masticatory muscle activity in healthy young adults. Journal of Craniomandibular Practice 20:91–98

Harper K A, Setchell D J 2002 The use of shimstock to access occlusal contacts: a laboratory study. International Journal of Prosthodontics; 15:347–352

Klineberg I J 1991 Occlusion: principles and assessment. Wright, Bristol

Lavigne G J, Goulet J-P, Zuconni M, Morrison F, Lobbezoo F 1999 Sleep disorders and the dental patient. An overview. Oral Surgery, Oral Medicine and Oral Pathology 88:257–272

Lobbezoo F, Naeije M 2001 Bruxism is mainly regulated centrally not peripherally. Review. Journal of Oral Rehabilitation 28:1085–1091

Millstein P, Maya A 2001 An evaluation of occlusal contact marking indicators. A descriptive quantitative method. Journal of the American Dental Association 132:1280–1286

Seligman D A, Pullinger A G 1995 The degree to which dental attrition in modern society is a function of age and of canine guidance. Journal of Orofacial Pain 9:266–275

Seligman D A, Pullinger A, Solberg W K 1988 The prevalence of dental attrition and its association with factors of age, gender, occlusion and TMJ symptomatology. Journal of Dental Research 67:1323–1333

Truelove E L, Sommers E E, LeResche L, Dworkin S F, von Korf M 1992 Clinical diagnostic criteria for TMD: new classification permits multiple diagnoses. Journal of the American Dental Association 123:47–54

Wänman A 1995 The relationship between muscle tenderness and craniomandibular disorders. A study of 35-year-olds from the general population. Journal of Orofacial Pain 9:235–243

Witter D J, Creugers N H, Kreulen Chiang Mai, de Haan A F 2001 Occlusal stability in shortened dental arches. Journal of Dental Research 80:432–436

Young W G 2002 The oral medicine of tooth wear. Australian Dental Journal 46:236–250

6

Articulators and evaluation of study casts

R. Jagger

Synopsis

Articulators are an essential component of restorative dentistry. When casts of a patient's dental arches are placed on an articulator they may be used to assess the dental occlusion and to allow formation of the occlusal surfaces of dental prostheses and indirect restorations.

There are many designs and each, to a greater or lesser extent, reproduces the relationship of a patient's maxilla to mandible during jaw movements.

This chapter describes the different types of articulators and describes how they are used to examine the occlusion.

Key points

- Articulators are described under the following headings:
  - **Simple hinge**
  - **Average value**
  - **Semiadjustable**
  - **Fully adjustable**
- Facebows and their application are described
- Occlusal records are an associated component of restorative dentistry. Their relevance to articulator systems is indicated
  - **Retruded jaw position (RP) or centric relation**
  - **Intercuspal contact position (ICP) or centric occlusion**
  - **Lateral and protrusive records**
  - **Dynamic records**
- Choosing an articulator

ARTICULATORS AND FACEBOW SYSTEMS

Articulators

An articulator is a hinged mechanical device to which maxillary and mandibular casts are attached, and which is intended to reproduce, to a greater or lesser extent, the relationship of a patient's maxilla to mandible in intercuspal contact position (ICP) and for lateral and protrusive jaw movements.

Articulators are used to:

- study the way the teeth occlude for diagnosis and treatment planning
- allow the formation of the occlusal surfaces during the laboratory preparation and adjustment of fixed and removable prostheses and indirect dental restorations.

There are many designs but in general there are four different types:

- simple hinge
- average value (plane-line)
- semi-adjustable
- fully adjustable.

Simple hinge articulators are capable of single hinge movement only and do not allow lateral movements (Fig. 6.1A). They are usually smaller than the patient's jaws and therefore intercuspal position recordings do not allow accurate articulation. They are consequently of very limited value.

Average value articulators have their condylar angle fixed at 30°. There is usually no provision for an adjustment for lateral mandibular shift. There is adjustable incisal guidance. These articulators represent an improvement on simple hinge articulators and may be considered to be sufficiently accurate for reproducing ICP on study casts (Fig. 6.1B).

Semi-adjustable articulators allow adjustment of condylar inclination and Bennett angle and sometimes for Bennett movement. Intercondylar width is usually fixed at 110 mm, but some articulators allow different intercondylar width settings.

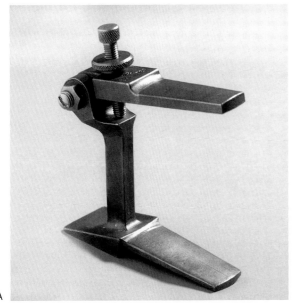

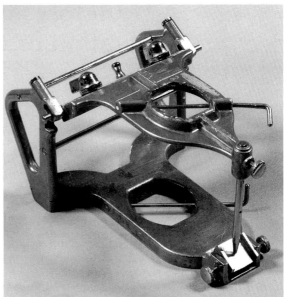

A   B

Fig. 6.1 **A** Hinge articulator. **B** Average value articulator.

These articulators may be either arcon or non-arcon in design (Fig. 6.2A–C). Arcon describes articulators in which the condylar mechanism is designed with the fossa box in the upper member of the articulator and the condylar sphere in the lower member of the articulator. This duplicates the anatomical arrangement of the temporomandibular (TM) joint. The arrangement allows distraction of the condyles in a similar manner to what is believed to occur in the TM joint.

The non-arcon articulators have a ball-and-slot mechanism in which the condylar ball is attached to the upper member and the slot mechanism to the lower member.

Condylar and Bennett angles are obtained from protrusive and lateral occlusal records (see below) or are set at average values.

Incisal guidance, the anterior guiding component of articulation, is simulated on the articulator by alteration of the angle of inclination of the incisal guidance table. The setting may be made by reference to the overbite and overjet relationship of the anterior teeth. If there is no existing guidance (where anterior teeth are absent), an average value can be set.

Custom-made incisal guidance tables of an existing incisal scheme can be made on an articulator using study casts.

Fully adjustable articulators are complex but allow closest duplication of the true clinical conditions. These articulators are designed to duplicate TM joint features by

a series of condylar adjustments and also allow curved translation paths (Fig. 6.2D–F).

The condylar settings may be determined by pantographic and stereographic records (see Figs 6.5 and 6.6).

Facebows

A *facebow* is an instrument that records the relationship of the maxilla to the hinge axis of rotation of the mandible. It allows the maxillary cast to be placed in an equivalent relationship on the articulator (Fig. 6.3).

In order to precisely identify the true hinge axis, it is necessary to use a *hinge axis locator* and then use a *hinge axis facebow*.

More commonly, facebows are used with an arbitrary hinge axis that is located at a point 12 mm along a line drawn from the upper aspect of the superior border of the tragus of the ear to the outer canthus of the eye. This point is used to position the condylar locator of the facebow. Alternatively, and now more commonly, the external ear canal is used with an ear facebow which provides an arbitrary point of reference for each TM joint. The geometric relationship of the ear canal to the TM joint is accommodated in the design of the facebow.

Facebows also allow transfer of intercondylar distance, which can be adjusted, on some articulators.

In dentate patients the facebow *fork* is used to locate the occlusal and incisal surfaces of the maxillary teeth. Wax or

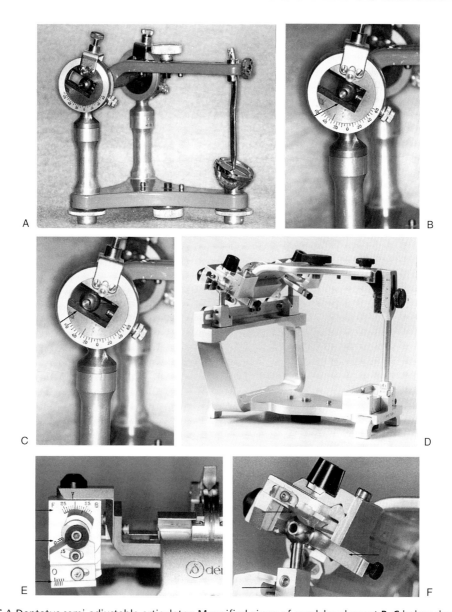

Fig. 6.2   A–C A Dentatus semi-adjustable articulator. Magnified views of condylar element **B**, **C** below show the 'ball and slot' mechanism. In the zero position the condylar sphere (arrowed) contacts the anterior stop; with a right lateral movement of the articulator the sphere moves distally along the slot (arrowed). This is a 'non-arcon' articulator where the condylar sphere is attached to the upper member. **D–F** A Denar D5A fully adjustable articulator. The condylar elements (arrowed) are different from those in **A**. This is an 'arcon' articulator where the condylar sphere is attached to the lower member, similarly to the anatomical arrangement in the skull. The magnified view (**E**) shows the superior aspect of the right condylar element, and identifies adjustments for the rear wall of the fossa box (upper arrow), the progressive side shift (middle arrow) and the immediate side shift (lower arrow). The magnified view (**F**) shows the anteroinferior view and identifies the superior wall of the fossa box (note its contour – upper arrow), the medial wall (middle arrow) and the intercondylar width adjustment (lower arrow). (From Klineberg 1991, with permission.)

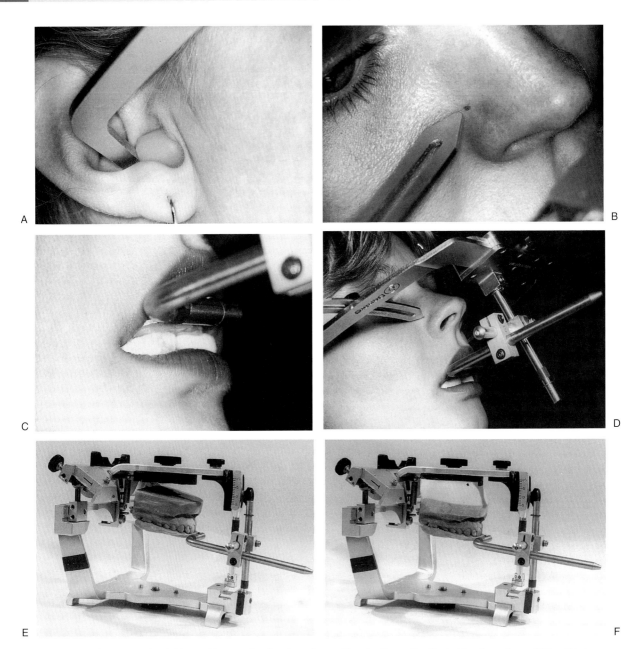

A

B

C

D

E

F

Fig. 6.3 Facebow transfer. **A** Ear rod locator for facebow in position in the patient's right external ear. **B** The third point of reference marker attached to a Slidematic facebow aligned with a mark placed on the side of the nose 43 mm above the incisal edge of tooth 1.1 or 2.1. **C** Facebow fork in position supported by cotton rolls against the mandibular teeth. **D** Slidematic facebow, fork and connecting jig in position. **E** A transfer fork, jig, and mounting block assembled on a Denar (MkII) articulator. **F** Maxillary cast attached to upper bow of articulator with mounting stone. (From Klineberg 1991, with permission.)

impression compound attached to the fork must locate the tooth cusps positively, but not extend into undercuts to avoid distortion. In edentulous patients the fork is attached to a maxillary occlusal rim.

Details of a technique using a Denar articulator and facebow that can be recommended are shown in Figure 6.3.

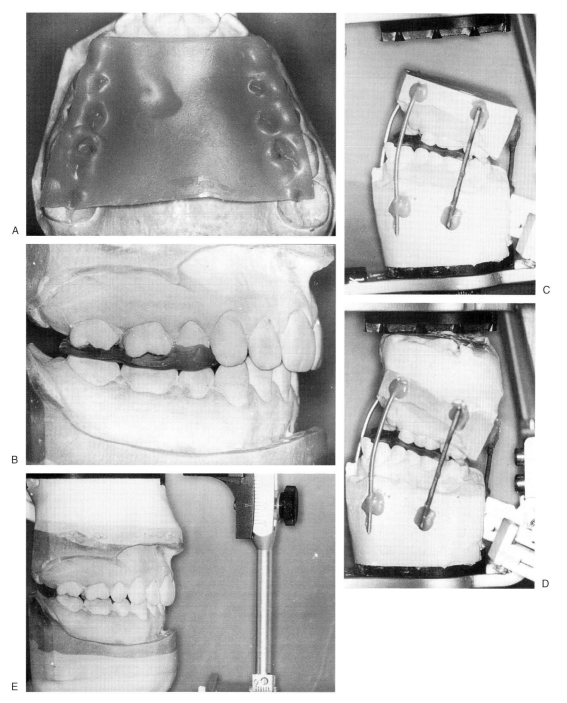

Fig. 6.4 Articulating mandibular cast. **A** Jaw record transfer on maxillary cast. **B** Jaw record transfer in place between maxillary and mandibular casts following trimming of excess wax. **C** Mandibular cast rigidly supported before mounting stone is added. **D** Mounting of mandibular cast – two-stage technique; first pour finishes just short of the mounting ring. **E** Mounting of mandibular cast completed. (From Klineberg 1991, with permission.)

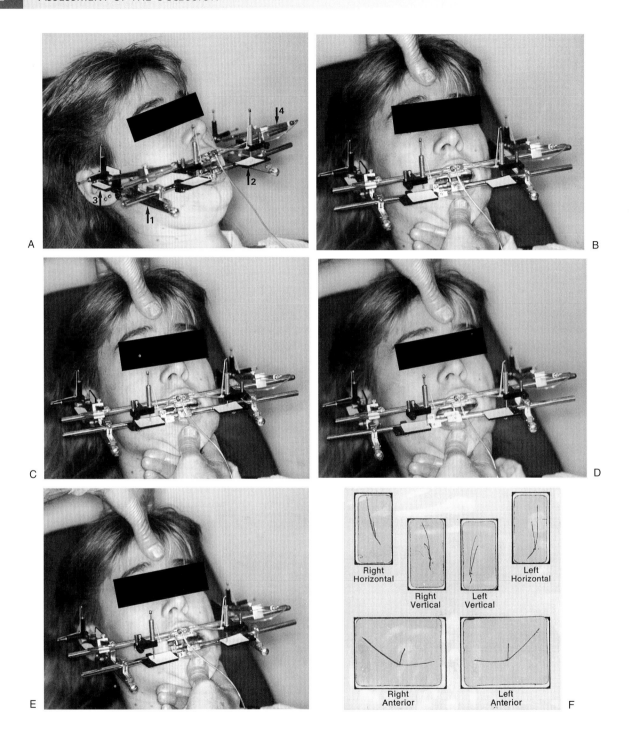

Fig. 6.5   Patient with a pantograph (Denar) attached to maxillary and mandibular intraoral clutches. **A** Note that the lower assembly (1) supports the two anterior horizontal tables (2) as well as the two posterior horizontal and two vertical tables (3). The upper assembly (4) contains six scribers which overlay the lower tables. Precut waxed paper recording blanks are placed on the tables. The scribers mark the blanks when the pantograph is activated and when the jaw is guided along the border paths to generate border path tracings. The system is pneumatically operated by compressed air and is remotely controlled by an on–off press-button switch. To activate the system, the button is depressed, the scribers contact the recording blanks and trace the movement generated with jaw guidance. **B** Gentle manual operator guidance establishing RP. **C** Gentle guidance while the patient performs a protrusive movement. Note markings on the anterior tables. **D** Gentle guidance of the jaw to the right. Note markings on the anterior tables and the position of the scribers. **E** Gentle guidance of the jaw to the left. Note markings on anterior tables, and the movement of the scribers in the opposite direction to their movement in **D**. **F** Pantographic tracings removed from the pantograph tables and placed on a storage sheet to be retained with the patient's records. A second recording made on another occasion may be compared with these recordings. (From Klineberg 1991, with permission.)

OCCLUSAL RECORDS

Retruded contact position (RCP) or centric relation (CR) record

This relation is used to articulate casts for diagnosis and treatment planning. The relation must be recorded with the teeth slightly apart in order to avoid any deflection by tooth contacts. RCP or CR is also used for complex, multiple restorations and for complete denture construction.

Details of a technique that can be recommended to record centric relation articulate casts are given in Figure 6.4.

Accurate study casts (silicone impressions)

- Trim a metal mesh to fit palatal aspect of the maxillary arch.
- Adapt mesh with hard wax to the palatal surfaces.
- Add two layers of a hard wax (for example, Alminax).
- Soften the wax on the mesh in hot water and place on the upper arch and then guide the mandible around the hinge axis so that the mandibular teeth indent but do not penetrate the wafer.
- Remove the wax wafer and add a very small amount of registration material (zinc oxide–eugenol paste is probably best).
- Replace the mesh and wafer in the mouth. Guide the mandible into the hinge position and allow the paste to set.
- Remove the record and verify by placing each cast in turn into its correct position.

Intercuspal contact position (ICP) or centric occlusion record

Casts can be articulated (or handheld) in this relationship of maximum tooth intercuspation for study purposes and if no change to the occlusal scheme is planned.

Lateral and protrusive records

These records are used to set the condylar angles of the articulator.

Recordings similar to that for centric relation may be taken but in required lateral or protrusive jaw positions. Alternatively, one of a number of graphical analysis systems which plot condylar inclination and allow measurement of Bennett movement and Bennett angle may be used. These systems require an upper and lower clutch attached to the upper and lower teeth to support and attach an upper and lower bow. The upper bow holds a grid on which the condylar movement details are marked, and the lower bow contains the measuring and marking rods. Once the system is attached, the hinge axis is determined and condylar inclination on jaw opening and Bennett movement and Bennett angle recorded during lateral border movements with gentle operator guidance of the jaw.

Dynamic records

Tracing plates

Single plane   Dynamic recordings of mandibular movements in a single plane can be made with tracing plates or acrylic moulding devices attached to intraoral clutches which are attached to the teeth. The acrylic clutches are thin plastic plates that engage undercuts of the teeth. The lower clutch has a central bearing pin that, during mandibular movements, engages the tracing plate on the inferior surface of the upper clutch. The tracing made on the plate when the mandible moves from centric relation to lateral border positions is known as the 'Gothic arch' tracing. The apex of the arch represents centric relation.

Pantographic tracings   The pantograph is a device used in conjunction with fully adjustable articulators that traces border paths of movement in three planes (Fig. 6.5).

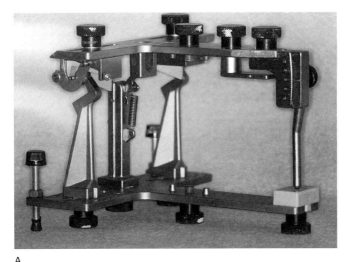

A

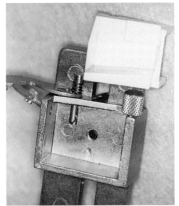

B

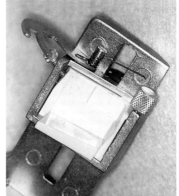

C

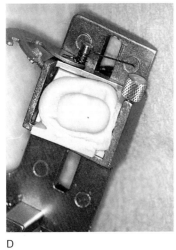

D

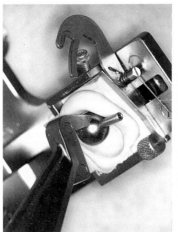

E

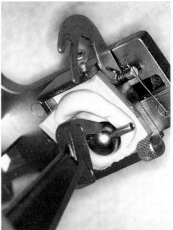

F

Fig. 6.6 Stereographic TM joint system. The stereographic articulator allows customised condylar fossa mouldings to be prepared individually for each patient. The mouldings incorporate the specific details of condylar movement. **A** TM joint fully adjustable arcon articulator. **B** Inferior view of the fossa box (metal) with the plastic insert above. The plastic insert supports the acrylic resin dough while moulding of fossa details is in progress. **C** Inferior view of the fossa box incorporating the plastic insert. **D** Inferior view of a moulded fossa. The condylar element has been removed to show the details of the fossa moulding (or condylar analogue). **E** Inferior view of the condylar element showing movement of the condylar sphere along the moulded fossa into a protrusive jaw position. **F** Inferior view of the condylar element showing the condylar sphere in the centric reference position in the moulded fossa analogue. (From Klineberg 1991, with permission.)

These tracings are used to set the articulator guidance mechanisms. Six tracing plates are attached to the mandibular clutch. Six tracing pins are attached to the maxillary clutch. When the mandible is manipulated to produce border movements the pins trace both horizontal and vertical tracings on the plates.

The traces allow determination of centric relation (from the Gothic arch) and degree and timing of Bennett movement.

Stereographic recording

Stereographic recordings (Fig. 6.6) are used with the TM joint articulator. They are three-dimensional recordings of mandibular movement that are made by moulding autopolymerising acrylic resin intraorally. In this case the mandibular clutch has a central bearing screw and the maxillary clutch has four cutting studs. Acrylic resin at the dough stage is placed onto the lower clutch at the location of the studs in the upper clutch. The patient is guided to border movements as the dough sets.

Once the acrylic resin has set, the jaw is guided through the border movements and the studs define the mouldings, forcing a precise record.

The record may then be transferred to the articulator, and the Gothic arch engraved by the studs allows the dentist/technician to make customised condylar mouldings, also in autopolymerising resin, within the right and left fossa box of the articulator.

CHOOSING AN ARTICULATOR

Simple hinge articulators

These articulators are of limited value in restorative dentistry and prosthodontics but may allow a preliminary evaluation of static tooth arrangement on study casts.

Average value articulators

These articulators produce an approximation of condylar movements and are frequently used to design and prepare complete dentures and simple restorations.

Semi-adjustable articulators

These articulators are recommended for most dental restorations.

The maxillary cast articulation with a facebow relates the maxillary cast to the condylar axis and allows a reasonable approximation of the arc of rotation of the jaw in centric relation. This also allows an increase of occlusal vertical dimension (OVD) by raising the height of the articulator pin, as the hinge axis is the same as the articulator axis of rotation.

Articulating the casts using an RCP (CR) record allows the examination of centric discrepancies. The decision whether to use an arcon or non-arcon articulator is largely a matter of operator preference. All semi-adjustable articulators are more accurate than plane line or simple hinge articulators but are less accurate than fully adjustable articulators.

Fully adjustable articulators

Fully adjustable articulators allow accurate replication of jaw relationships and lateral and protrusive jaw mandibular movement. They are complex instruments that are technique-sensitive. Their use is principally in extensive fixed prosthodontics and restorative dentistry.

OCCLUSAL ASSESSMENT AND STUDY CAST ANALYSIS

Good quality casts must be mounted on a semi-adjustable articulator using a facebow and a centric relation record. Condylar settings may be adjusted using lateral and protrusive records.

Verification of accuracy of articulation of casts

It is important to ensure that the articulated casts accurately reproduce the situation in the patient's mouth, as there are several causes of errors in articulation. Common errors are incorrect occlusal record, inaccurate casts and mounting errors.

Occlusal assessment

The following procedure can be recommended for detailed analysis of occlusal contacts.

Using ultrafine GMH foils and Artus shimstock, analyse tooth contacts on articulated casts in the following sequence:

1. Determine RP stops (if RP stops are absent on posterior teeth, use the verification record to check that the articulation is correct).
2. Locate the position of plunger cusps.
3. Determine the presence of any slide from RP to IP and its dimensions: vertical, lateral, anteroposterior.
4. Check the stability of supporting cusps and intercuspal stops in RP and IP.
5. Examine whether there are marginal ridge discrepancies and whether affected teeth have stable opposing contacts.

6. Move the casts into protrusive and lateral excursions to determine whether there is canine protection (guidance) or group function.
7. Examine whether there are working-side or non-working interferences.
8. If using an arcon type articulator, note any condylar displacement from IP to RP.

References

Klineberg I J 1991 Occlusion: principles and assessment. Wright, Bristol.

Further reading

Baetz K, Klineberg I J 1986 An analysis of stereographic jaw recording techniques. Australian Dental Journal 31: 117–123

Cabot L B 1998 Using articulators to enhance clinical practice. British Dental Journal 184: 272–276

Celenza F V 1979 An analysis of articulators. Dental Clinics of North America 23: 305–326

Clayton J A, Kotowicz W E, Zahler J M 1976 Pantographic tracings of mandibular movements and occlusion. Journal of Prosthetic Dentistry 25: 389–396

Hobo S, Shillingburg H T, Whitsett L D 1976 Articulation for restorative dentistry. Journal of Prosthetic Dentistry 36:35–43

Lundeen H C, Shyrock E F Gibbs C H 1978 An evaluation of mandibular border movements: their character and significance. Journal of Prosthetic Dentistry 40: 442–452

CLINICAL PRACTICE AND THE OCCLUSION

7 Temporomandibular joint disorders

G. Carlsson

Synopsis

This chapter presents a brief review of the most common temporomandibular (TM) joint disorders, with an emphasis on their association with dental occlusion. The evidence for an occlusal aetiology of TM joint disorders is weak, whereas it is well established that several TM joint disorders can cause occlusal disturbances. The TM joint disorders presented comprise disc interference and traumatic disorders, osteoarthritis and rheumatoid arthritis, and other less frequent disorders. A careful history and a clinical examination, including imaging of the TM joint, will in most cases be sufficient for a preliminary diagnosis. Many patients with benign TM joint disorders can be managed in general dental practice, whereas others will require specialist and multidisciplinary diagnosis and treatment.

Key points

- Many diseases may involve the TM joints. The most common and the most studied are osteoarthrosis and rheumatoid arthritis, as well as disc interference disorders
- It is often claimed that occlusal disturbances can cause TM joint disorders, but the evidence for that is weak. On the other hand, it is well established that several disorders affecting the TM joints may cause occlusal disturbances (for example, occlusal instability and/or anterior open bite in patients with rheumatoid arthritis)
- Disc displacement is considered to be the most common TM joint disorder. It involves

a dysfunction of the condyle–disc relation, but the disc position is either not at all or only weakly related to clinical symptoms

- Disc displacement disorders can usually be managed with a conservative approach, and more 'aggressive' methods are seldom indicated
- Several traumatic TM joint disorders are associated with changes in occlusion, which require careful consideration in diagnosis and treatment
- Osteoarthrosis is a degeneration of the TM joint but is in general a benign disorder with minor or no symptoms and a good prognosis. In osteoarthritis an inflammatory component is added to the joint degeneration. Acute inflammatory phases associated with pain and dysfunction are usually reversible with simple treatment
- A substantial proportion of patients with rheumatoid arthritis may have TM joint involvement. TM joint involvement is related to the severity and duration of the systemic disease. About 10% of patients with rheumatoid arthritis are afflicted with severe occlusal disturbances and dysfunction of the masticatory system
- There is often a poor correlation between findings from TM joint imaging and clinical signs and symptoms of TM joint disorders
- Investigation of a patient with a possible TM joint disorder may include a history and various clinical, laboratory and imaging procedures; however, in most cases the history and a clinical examination of the masticatory system focusing on TM joint mobility, sounds and tenderness to palpation may be sufficient for a preliminary diagnosis and initial treatment

INTRODUCTION

The role played by disorders of the TM joint in producing signs and symptoms in temporomandibular disorders (TMDs) has been much discussed. In the early development of concepts of TMD, TM joint problems were the focus. Interest then turned to the musculature as the most frequent source of pain and dysfunction of the masticatory system. During the 1980s many clinicians thought that internal derangements of the TM joint were the most prevalent factor in TMDs. Today it is generally accepted that TMDs include a variety of different disorders involving the TM joint and the muscles of mastication, separately or together (Carlsson & Magnusson 1999). To classify TMDs either as arthrogenous or myogenous is difficult, because patients with a primary joint disorder usually have secondary muscle dysfunction, and patients with a primary muscle disorder may exhibit joint symptoms (Stegenga 2001).

More than 100 different diseases can affect the musculoskeletal system and many of these may also involve the TM joint. Some of these are rare and of limited interest for the general dental practitioner, but a few are relatively common, such as osteoarthrosis/osteoarthritis (OA) and rheumatoid arthritis (RA), and the dentist should be familiar with them.

In this chapter we will focus on TM joint disorders that in various ways may be associated with changes in occlusion.

DISC INTERFERENCE DISORDERS

Variations from the textbook appearance of the TM joint disc have been termed disc displacements and they may occur in various directions, anterior displacements probably being most frequent (Fig. 7.1). Several descriptions

have been presented over the years but the following classification is probably the most frequently cited:

- disc displacement with reduction (the displaced disc reduces on opening, usually resulting in a noise, clicking; this is called reciprocal clicking when the noise is heard during both the opening and closing movement)
- disc displacement without reduction, with limited opening
- disc displacement without reduction, without limited opening.

The symptoms described in association with such disc interference disorders vary greatly, but usually include pain, tenderness to palpation of joints and/or muscles, joint sounds and reduced mobility. There does not appear to be any close correlation between the structural variation of the disc–condyle complex and clinical symptomatology; some patients with verified 'disc displacement' may lack symptoms, and others who have symptoms and disc displacement may improve without change of the structural TM joint findings.

The aetiology is not well understood but trauma and general joint hypermobility are frequently reported in the histories of patients with disc interference disorders.

Management

During the 1980s there was an enormous increase in interest in disc interference disorders. This resulted in a rapid improvement of diagnostic and therapeutic methods, but it also probably led to overdiagnosis and overtreatment (for example, use of magnetic resonance imaging (MRI), anterior positioning appliances followed by occlusal therapy, and various surgical methods), higher cost and sometimes increased risk for the patients. It has been repeatedly shown that many patients with TM joint disc displacement respond well to conservative treatment (Carlsson & Magnusson 1999). It is also well established that painless jaw function is possible with the disc displaced (Stegenga 2001). In the majority of patients diagnosed with disc interference disorders, the simple treatment modalities suggested previously for TMD patients should first be tried, that is, counselling/reassurance, medication and physical therapy, often including an interocclusal appliance. This conservative approach has proven effective according to long-term clinical follow-up investigations. In a sample of 40 patients with permanent disc displacement followed for 2.5 years without treatment, spontaneous improvement was observed in about 75% of the cases (Kurita et al 1998).

The use of protrusive positioning splints in order to 'capture the disc' is rarely indicated, as it may lead to serious changes in the occlusion, requiring extensive

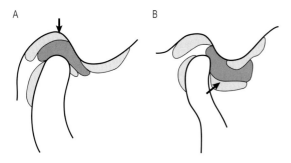

Fig. 7.1 Schematic drawings from arthrographic radiographs of TM joints. **A** Normal position of the disc. **B** Anteriorly displaced disc (arrow). (From Carlsson & Magnusson 1999, with permission.)

occlusal therapy. Some authors have even maintained that such treatment was worse than the 'disease' itself. Manipulation techniques to normalise the disc position in patients with disc displacement without reduction may be successful if the 'closed lock' is acute, that is, of short duration (Carlsson & Magnusson 1999).

A variety of surgical procedures have been applied and maintained to give good results when severe pain and dysfunction continued in association with disc interference disorders. However, long-term studies are lacking, as are randomised prospective studies. Surgery is certainly not the first method of choice.

It can be concluded that the rapid progress in TM joint imaging techniques made it clear that internal derangements (mechanical joint disorders of which disc displacements are only one) are more prevalent than previously thought. Today it is more and more accepted, however, that visualisation of the disc by methods such as arthrography and MRI result in an overemphasis on the mechanical aspects of disc displacement. Several studies have shown that disc position does not correlate well with pain or dysfunction; for example, approximately 30% of asymptomatic subjects received a radiographic or MRI diagnosis of 'disc displacement' (Stegenga 2001). The frequently used term 'disc displacement' has therefore been considered 'flawed because it implies the need for treatment'.

A careful history and a clinical examination, without use of sophisticated imaging techniques, and conservative management should be adequate for most patients with disc interference disorders. If severe pain and dysfunction remain after such an approach, the patient is best referred to a specialist clinic.

TRAUMATIC TM JOINT DISORDERS

Injury to the TM joint may result from internal forces (such as from jaw muscles) or from external forces (such as contact sport or a slamming door) applied to the joint area or along the mandible. Such trauma may produce damage to the soft tissues, the condyle or both. The consequences may be joint dislocation, haemarthrosis and condylar fracture.

Acute dislocation

Diagnosis and treatment of an acute dislocation should be familiar to all dentists: the patient cannot close the mouth and there is an anterior open bite ('open lock'). In front of one or both auditory canals there is a depression, before which it is usually possible to palpate the condyle positioned anterior to the articular eminence (Fig. 7.2). When the dislocation is acute, reduction can often be done

without anaesthesia, by bimanual manipulation of the mandible from its open locked position. A classical description suggests the following procedure: the operator stands in front of the patient and use the thumbs to apply pressure to the molar regions in a downward direction; at the same time the chin is raised with the other fingers, after which the mandible is forced backwards. If the dislocation occurred a day or days previously, there may be considerable pain and muscular tension. In such cases, local anaesthetic blocks of the TM joint area(s) are performed before the manipulation, to provide patient comfort and reduction of muscle guarding. In rare cases, especially after longstanding dislocation, intravenous sedation or even general anaesthesia may be necessary to enable manipulation of the dislocated joint. After a successful mandibular reduction the patient should be advised to avoid wide opening movements and heavy chewing for several days to a week.

Haemarthrosis

A blow to the mandible or extensive stretching of the joint's soft tissues may lead to oedema or haemorrhage within the joint space. When the trauma has not led to mandibular fracture the patient will usually present with mild swelling and tenderness in the TM joint area, pain

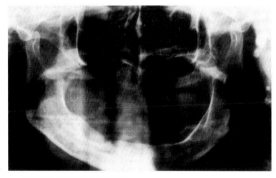

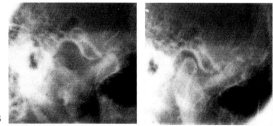

Fig. 7.2 Acute dislocation of the TM joints. **A** Panoramic radiograph of a bilateral dislocation. Both condyles are anterior to the articular eminences. **B** Transcranial radiograph of the dislocated right TM joint of the patient in **A**. **C** The right TM joint after reduction.

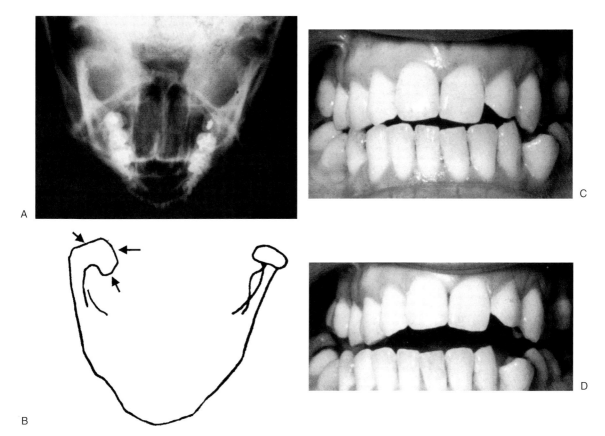

A

B

C

D

Fig. 7.3 Condylar fracture with an inward dislocation of the condyle. **A** Axial radiograph. **B** Tracing of the radiograph in **A**. **C** Maximum intercuspal position and **D** retruded contact position in a patient who had a unilateral condylar fracture a few months previously.

on movement and reduced joint mobility. The patient often reports that the teeth on the injured side do not fit, which is the clinical manifestation of the lateral open bite caused by the effusion and haemarthrosis within the joint space. This can be seen radiographically as an increased distance between the condyle and the fossa. This condition is sometimes referred to as *traumatic arthritis*.

If the tissue injury is not severe, the acute symptoms usually disappear within one or a few weeks. Ice may be applied intermittently to skin overlying the joint area during the first day, after which massage and careful jaw exercises may be introduced gradually to normalise joint mobility. If pain and swelling are severe, drugs with analgesic and antiphlogistic effect may be prescribed. It is important to avoid occlusal therapy during the acute phase, as the occlusion will normalise when the joint effusion resolves.

Condylar fractures

Condylar and subcondylar fractures comprise a substantial part of all mandibular fractures. Patients will typically present with an open bite and a slight mandibular shift toward the affected side. With bilateral condyle fractures there is an anterior open bite. Patients with such fractures usually require specialist evaluation and treatment. However, the sequelae of condylar fractures on the occlusion are of general interest. In children with condyle fractures, the great capacity for TM joint remodelling results in only minor or no long-term effects on the occlusion. In adults, occlusal instability, including an increased distance between the retruded and the intercuspal jaw positions, is a frequent consequence of a previous condylar fracture (Fig. 7.3). This requires special consideration in diagnosis of the occlusion for prosthodontic rehabilitation.

OSTEOARTHROSIS/OSTEOARTHRITIS

Degenerative joint disease is the most common form of rheumatoid disease affecting the human body. There are several synonymous terms used for this disease, osteoarthrosis and osteoarthritis being the most frequent. It has been suggested that osteoarthritis be used for disorders with clinical symptoms (indicating an ongoing inflammatory process), and osteoarthrosis where inflammation is absent or minimal and the patient is asymptomatic. Others maintain that this disorder involves both degeneration and inflammation and that osteoarthritis is the logical term (Stegenga 2001). It can be practical to use the abridged form OA for both.

OA is primarily non-inflammatory in nature, with initial involvement of the cartilaginous and subchondral layers of the joint. It is defined as a degenerative condition of the joint, characterised by fibrillation and deterioration of the articular tissue, and concomitant changes in the form of the articular components (Zarb & Carlsson 1999). The first changes in the articular tissues in OA are rarely visible radiographically. Radiographic evidence of changes in form will typically appear only after considerable time, which can explain the poor correlation between clinical and radiographic signs of OA. It is often a gradual non-symptomatic development of OA, but the superimposition of secondary inflammatory changes, synovitis, can cause transitory clinical symptoms. The long-term outcome of OA of the TM joint is, in general, good.

Epidemiology

Population studies have shown that OA is an extremely common joint disorder but the prevalence varies in different joints, even if it is strongly correlated with increasing age. The reported prevalence of OA in the TM joint varies widely in several studies, probably for methodological reasons. It appears safe to conclude that TM joint OA increases with age, and it is more frequent in women than in men, for ages above 50 years, as is also the case in other joints of the body (Zarb & Carlsson 1999).

Aetiology

Even if overloading has been proposed to be a major aetiologic factor, it is prudent to recognise that the understanding of the aetiology of OA is far from complete. The literature does not contain compelling evidence for an occlusal contribution to TMDs and this is true also for OA of the TM joint (Zarb & Carlsson 1999; Pullinger & Seligman 2000). It has been suggested that OA represents an organ failure due to an imbalance between the normal tissue turnover of synthesis and breakdown. A relative increase of breakdown/degenerative activity leads to accumulation of degradative products resulting in an inflammatory response. The often-proposed relationship between disc displacement and OA has recently been questioned, as no strong evidence is available. Present research focuses more on the microscopic and molecular level of joint tissues rather than disc displacement (see Ch. 4) (Stegenga 2001).

Diagnosis

The signs and symptoms are very similar to those of the neuromuscular type of TMD. However, there are some features that might help differential diagnosis:

- They are almost always unilateral.
- Symptoms often worsen during the day.
- Pain is located in the joint itself.
- Crepitation is a more common joint sound than clicking (but it is a late sign of the disorder).
- Radiographic changes of the TM joint are frequent (for example, condyle flattening, osteophytes, sclerosis, decreased joint space).

It is important to realise that there is often poor correlation between clinical and radiographic findings and many subjects with a radiographic diagnosis of OA may be asymptomatic or reveal only crepitus (Fig. 7.4). Laboratory findings in synovial fluid have shown promising results in identifying markers of disease activity. The methods offer interesting research possibilities but are not yet applicable to OA diagnosis in general dental practice (Zarb & Carlsson 1999).

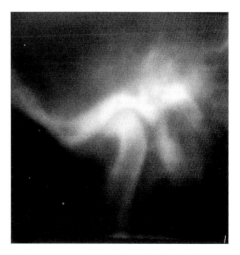

Fig. 7.4 Tomogram of the left TM joint with extensive deformation indicating OA. The patient had a short period of pain and dysfunction but functioned well for many years both before and after that event.

Patients with OA were characterised by a longer slide between the retruded contact position (RCP) and intercuspal position (ICP), larger overjet and reduced overbite. These occlusal characteristics were interpreted to be the consequence of articular remodelling associated with OA, rather than its cause (Pullinger & Seligman 2000).

OA often has acute and chronic stages. It has been estimated that the average duration of the acute painful stage is 9–12 months. The disease process tends to 'burn out', and the TM joint often shows extensive osseous changes but surprisingly good function. The diagnosis of OA must acknowledge the usually favourable long-term prognosis of this mainly benign disorder.

Management

Because of the current knowledge of the favourable prognosis of OA, the first step in treatment is to reassure the patient about the problems associated with this benign disorder. For patients with only crepitus or mild symptoms, reassurance is the only treatment necessary. For patients with more severe symptoms, including pain and dysfunction, treatment may include one or more of the following:

- medication (most frequently non-steroidal anti-inflammatory drugs (NSAIDs) but sometimes, in cases of severe pain, intra-articular injection of glucocorticoid
- physical therapy (rest and soft diet in the most acute stage, gradually beginning jaw exercises when pain subsides, to promote normal mandibular function)
- splint therapy – interocclusal stabilisation appliance (to provide reduction of a possible overloading of the joint structures).

Surgery is very seldom indicated in the treatment of TM joint OA.

RHEUMATOID ARTHRITIS

Rheumatoid arthritis (RA) is a systemic inflammatory disease, that involves peripheral joints in a symmetric distribution. The aetiology of RA is still largely unknown but immunological mechanisms appear to play an important role. The prevalence of RA has been reported to be about 1–2% of the adult population, with incidence figures of 0.03–0.1% per year. RA has shown a 3:1 female predilection. TM joint involvement in patients with RA depends on the duration and severity of the systemic disease, but it can be expected that about half of them will develop TM joint complaints (Carlsson & Magnusson 1999). Severe forms of the disease with significant functional disability, including major occlusal disturbances, occur in 10–15% of these patients.

Diagnosis

Diagnosing RA of the TM joint will seldom present problems, as the systemic disease usually starts in other joints before the TM joint and the diagnosis has most probably been established when the TM joint is affected. Symptoms include pain at rest and on chewing, stiffness in the morning, and difficulty in opening the mouth. As the disease process continues, the stability of the occlusion is often destroyed, revealed as an unstable intercuspal position and an increased distance between RCP and ICP. Anterior bite opening may occur due to destruction of the condyles (Fig. 7.5). Radiographic changes include erosion of the cortical contour of the joint components, reduced joint space, subchondral cysts and gradually severe destruction of the bone, eventually leading to complete loss of the condyle. Modern diagnostic methods such as analysis of TM joint fluid, laboratory tests, thermologic and arthroscopic techniques have improved our knowledge of the disease, but they are limited to specialist clinics. There is good evidence that neuropeptides take part in the modulation of TM joint arthritis and pain (Zarb & Carlsson 1999).

Treatment

Because RA is a systemic disease, a physician must manage the primary care, while the dentist can take part in management of local TM joint signs and symptoms. This usually involves supportive therapy to reduce pain, inflammation and excessive joint loading (Carlsson & Magnusson 1999).

Pain in an acute phase is most probably associated with inflammation and therefore analgesics with anti-inflammatory effects should be prescribed, for example, acetylsalicylic acid or NSAIDs such as naproxen or ibuprofen. If the pain is severe, intra-articular injection of a glucocorticosteroid often gives rapid relief.

When the acute pain has subsided or when there are only minor symptoms, physical exercises are indicated to improve joint muscle function and strength. Positive short- and long-term effects of physical training in TM joint RA-patients have been shown in a comparative study.

The role played by occlusal factors in the development of RA of the TM joint is uncertain. From a clinical point of view it is recommended, however, to provide all patients with RA with a stable occlusion, for example, by eliminating gross occlusal interferences, restoring lost teeth by means of (provisional) prosthetic appliances or temporarily with interocclusal appliances. An anterior open bite caused by RA can often be reduced by simple occlusal adjustment. If the disease has resulted in a very severe malocclusion, orthognathic surgery may be indicated.

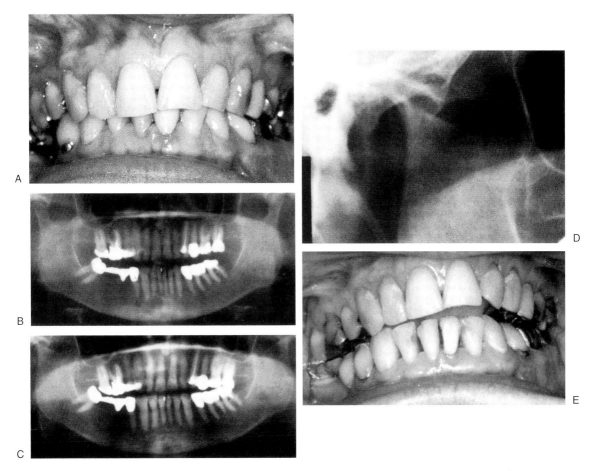

Fig. 7.5 Patient with rheumatoid arthritis. **A** Maximum intercuspal position before any involvement of the TM joints has occurred. **B** Panoramic radiograph after about 10 years when the TM joints start to be involved. **C** Panoramic radiograph 3 years later when severe destruction of the TM joints has occurred. **D** Part of the radiograph in **C** showing an almost total loss of the condyle. **E** Maximum intercuspal position showing an anterior open bite and occlusal instability at the time of radiographs **C** and **D**.

A problem in prosthodontic rehabilitation of patients with RA is the continuing joint destruction that may disturb occlusal stability of any reconstruction. A check of the disease activity can be obtained from the rheumatologist, and long-term provisional prostheses may be necessary if acute phases can still be expected. Another problem is the often substantially increased distance between the retruded and habitual occlusal positions. The retruded position cannot be used as a reference for transfer records because the disease processes have destroyed the joint structures. A more anterior position that is comfortable for the patient and acceptable to the musculature is chosen.

OTHER TM JOINT DISORDERS

The TM joint may also be afflicted in many other systemic diseases; for example, psoriatic arthritis, ankylosing spondylitis, gout and acromegaly. The prevalence of TM joint involvement in these diseases is not well known but several of them can lead to changes in the dental occlusion. An example is acromegaly, which is a chronic disease of adults caused by hypersecretion of growth hormone leading to enlargement of many parts of the skeleton, including the mandible and the TM joints (Fig. 7.6). The importance of including questions on general health in the patient's history is obvious.

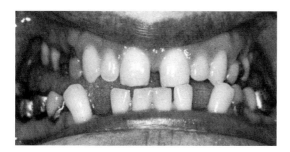

Fig. 7.6 In a patient with acromegaly, the extensive growth of the mandible has led to loss of all occlusal contacts.

Neoplasms may be found in the TM joint. Malignant tumours are extremely rare, and when they occur they are most often metastatic. Since it has been reported that they may present with symptoms similar to TMDs, patients with a history of cancer and TM joint dysfunction must be referred for a radiographic examination of the TM joint. More common, but still very rare, are benign neoplasms, which may change the form of the joint components and cause dysfunction and occlusal disturbances. Although not a neoplasm but a developmental disturbance, unilateral condylar hyperplasia is associated with similar consequences, due to the enlarged condyle, which will also lead to facial asymmetry and malocclusion.

 References

Carlsson G E, Magnusson T 1999 Management of temporomandibular disorders in the general dental practice. Quintessence, Chicago

Kurita K, Westesson P L, Yuasa H et al 1998 Natural course of untreated symptomatic temporomandibular disc displacement without reduction. Journal of Dental Research 77:361–365

Pullinger A G, Seligman D A 2000 Quantification and validation of predictive values of occlusal variables in temporomandibular disorders using a multifactorial analysis. Journal of Prosthetic Dentistry 83:66–75

Stegenga B 2001 Osteoarthritis of the temporomandibular joint organ and its relationship to disc displacement. Journal of Orofacial Pain 15:193–205

Zarb G A, Carlsson G E 1999 Temporomandibular disorders: osteoarthritis. Journal of Orofacial Pain 13:295–306

 Further reading

Backe M, Zak M, Jensen B L, Pedersen F K, Kreiborg S 2001 Orofacial pain, jaw function, and temporomandibular disorders in women with a history of juvenile chronic arthritis or persistent juvenile chronic arthritis. Oral Surgery, Oral Medicine, Oral Pathology, Oral Radiolology and Endodontics 92:406–414

De Boever J A, Carlsson G E 1996 Temporomandibular disorders and the need for prosthetic treatment. In: Öwall B, Käyser A F, Carlsson G E (eds) Prosthodontics: principles and management strategies. Mosby-Wolfe, London

De Boever J A, Carlsson G E, Klineberg I J 2000 Need for occlusal therapy and prosthodontic treatment in the management of temporomandibular disorders. Part II: Tooth loss and prosthodontic treatment. Journal of Oral Rehabilitation 27:647–659

Holmlund A B, Axelsson S, Gynther G W 2001 A comparison of discectomy and arthroscopic lysis and lavage for the treatment of chronic closed lock of the temporomandibular joint: a randomized outcome study. Journal of Oral and Maxillofacial Surgery 59:972–977

Kopp S 2001 Neuroendocrine, immune, and local responses related to temporomandibular disorders. Journal of Orofacial Pain 15:9–28

Minakuchi H, Kuboki T, Matsuka Y et al 2001 Randomized controlled evaluation of non-surgical treatments for temporomandibular joint anterior disc displacement without reduction. Journal of Dental Research 80:924–928

Okesson J P (ed) 1996 Orofacial pain. Guidelines for assessment, diagnosis and management. Quintessence, Chicago.

Svensson B, Adell R, Kopp S 2000 Temporomandibular disorders in juvenile chronic arthritis patients. A clinical study. Swedish Dental Journal 24:83–92

Zarb G A, Carlsson G E, Sessle B J, Mohl N D 1994 Temporomandibular joint and masticatory muscle disorders. Munksgaard, Copenhagen

8 Jaw muscle disorders

M. Bakke

Synopsis

This chapter will review the current knowledge of the aetiology and physiology of jaw muscle disorders, and present an approach for their clinical assessment and treatment.

Jaw muscle disorders are characterised by pain that is usually aggravated by function, and by a limited range of jaw movement. They are present in 75% of patients with temporomandibular disorders (TMDs), and women are affected more frequently than men. Several contributing factors must be present for the development of jaw muscle disorders. No studies have yet fully explained the relative importance of potential risk factors.

The masseter and medial pterygoid muscles serve primarily as sources of power, while the temporalis and lateral pterygoid muscles are important for jaw stability. Overuse in terms of sustained activity and high-level contractions without rest periods is associated with raised intramuscular pressure, and leads to local ischaemia, increased membrane permeability, oedema and eventually cellular damage.

Muscle pain is generally described as a continuous deep dull ache or tightness or pressure. The onset is normally gradual, and may vary from a feeling of tiredness to a more severe sharp pain. The pain may result from trauma, sustained or forceful contractions, stretching or ischaemia. Local conditions, such as inflammation, increase the receptivity of the pain receptors, lowering their threshold for activation.

A comprehensive evaluation of the jaw muscles includes a systematic history and clinical examination. The clinical examination has two main purposes: to assess jaw function, and, if possible, to provoke the patient's pain. The treatment of jaw muscle disorders is directed towards reducing pain and improving function; it should generally be reversible, evidence-based, or at least based on well-established clinical practice.

Key points

- Jaw muscle disorders are a collection of conditions affecting the muscles, primarily characterised by pain and limited jaw movements; they are part of TMDs
- The primary masticatory muscles are the temporalis, masseter, and medial and lateral pterygoid muscles. The trigeminal nerve innervates the jaw muscles, and muscle fibres associated with long contraction times and resistance to fatigue predominate. The jaw muscles and the bite force adapt to the prevailing level of activity. There may be fibrosis with overuse
- The experience of muscle pain is poorly localised, but pain provoked by manual palpation more accurately identifies pain location. The intensity may be assessed by visual analogue scales (VASs) and by rating of the response to the palpation
- Limited mandibular opening, (less than 40 mm) is assessed by measurement in the incisor region, adding the amount of overbite or subtracting the amount of open bite
- Chronic localised myalgia in terms of myofascial pain is the most frequent jaw muscle disorder. Myofascial pain from jaw muscles may also be diagnosed as tension-type headache, and it may be secondary to disc displacements, osteoarthritis and rheumatoid arthritis of the temporomandibular (TM) joints

> • Counselling, analgesics and non-steroidal anti-inflammatory drugs (NSAIDs), physical therapy and intraoral appliances are the main treatments for jaw muscle disorders

EPIDEMIOLOGY AND AETIOLOGY OF JAW MUSCLE DISORDERS

Jaw muscle disorders, a collection of muscle conditions, are part of TMDs affecting TM joints and jaw muscles. Jaw muscle disorders are characterised by pain and limited jaw movements that are usually aggravated by function. According to studies using the Research Diagnostic Criteria (RDC) for TMD defined by Dworkin and LeResche (1992), muscle disorders are frequently found in TMDs, that is, in about 75% of the patients, whereas disc displacement disorders and disorders of arthralgia, arthritis and arthrosis are present in about 30% of the patients. Women are affected about twice as frequently as men, and the condition is most prevalent in young to middle-aged adults.

Pain in the jaw muscles, experienced as facial pain and headache, is the most prominent chronic pain condition in the orofacial region. Epidemiological studies indicate that about 5% of the population suffers from jaw muscle pain (myalgia) that is sufficiently severe to require treatment (Kuttila et al 1998), but there is considerable fluctuation in the presence and intensity of the pain. As in other musculoskeletal conditions, jaw muscle disorders often run a recurrent or chronic course, and there may be psychological factors that can either produce or influence the pain experience. Depression, which has been shown to be present in some TMD patients, as well as multiple pain conditions, increase the risk of the development of persistent pain. However, symptoms may also be transient, and spontaneous pain reduction may occur.

The aetiology of jaw muscle disorders is considered to be multifactorial, whereby several contributing factors must be present for a jaw muscle disorder to develop. No studies have yet fully explained the relative importance of potential risk factors, and there is presently no consensus of simple cause–effect relationships, for example, between occlusal features or specific jaw muscle activities and jaw muscle pain. Based on present information, only anterior open bite represents a true occlusal risk factor for myalgia (Pullinger & Seligman 2000), even if occlusal parameters have been shown to influence jaw muscle activity. Nocturnal bruxism has also been cited as being an important factor for development of myalgia, but in reality a certain amount of nocturnal bruxism is observed in most asymptomatic adults. Nocturnal bruxism is now

regarded as being a sleep disorder (Lobbezoo & Naeije 2001). Reduced jaw muscle strength (bite force) in patients with TMDs may represent a risk factor, but this reduction may also arise as a result of local pain.

Because of the unclear aetiology of jaw muscle disorders, there is no objective diagnostic method to easily differentiate the condition; there is no gold standard (such as tissue biopsy) against which a diagnostic test can be compared with accuracy and reliability. The best approach is a comprehensive medical and dental history and a comprehensive clinical examination.

PHYSIOLOGY AND FUNCTIONAL ANATOMY OF THE JAW MUSCLES

Knowledge of the anatomy and function of jaw muscles, as well as their typical features, should help with differential diagnoses of jaw muscle disorders.

Physiology

This section complements the comprehensive reviews of jaw muscle control and jaw movements in Chapter 2.

Jaw function during biting, mastication, swallowing and speech is determined by a complex interaction between jaw muscles, TM joints, teeth and the nervous system. The primary jaw muscles are the temporalis, masseter, and medial and lateral pterygoids. Branches from the mandibular nerve, external carotid artery and internal jugular vein innervate and vascularise the jaw muscles. The masseter and medial pterygoid muscles serve primarily as sources of power, while the temporalis and lateral pterygoid muscles are important for jaw stability. The jaw muscles function in concert with the suprahyoid and the infrahyoid muscles, supplemented by the tongue, lip and cheek muscles. The cervical muscles also have an indirect role through stabilising and changing head posture during mandibular movements (Eriksson et al 2000).

Muscle bulk is maintained by physical activity as well as naturally derived steroids and growth hormones. Inactivity leads to hypotrophy and training to hypertrophy, with changes in the diameter of muscle fibres. The muscle enzymes responsible for energy release during aerobic and anaerobic muscular effort, and the number of capillaries, adapt to the prevailing level of activity. Jaw muscles appear to have different tasks and functional activities from limb muscles because the capillary supply is better and the muscle fibre characteristics are different. In jaw muscles, fibres associated with long contraction times (slow twitch) and resistance to fatigue (type I) predominate. Overuse in terms of sustained activity and high level contractions without rest periods is associated with raised intramuscular pressure, and leads to local ischaemia, increased membrane permeability, oedema, and eventually cellular damage. In addition, slight post-exercise oedema and hyperaemia are seen, even after the chewing of gum, in healthy jaw muscles. It has been proposed that low jaw muscle strength might predispose to overuse. With breakdown of muscle tissue, fibrosis may take place, as well as possible regeneration of muscle fibres from satellite cells ('resting' myoblasts), which also contribute to muscle growth.

The mandibular elevators, especially the temporalis and the masseter, are the larger jaw muscles. Their level of activity contributes to bite force, and is influenced by muscle thickness and fibre size and distribution. Bite force is greater in men than in women, but is also dependent on age and occlusal contacts. There is a correlation between the bite force and facial morphology, as the vertical facial relationship and jaw angle decrease with increasing strength; thus weak elevator muscles appear to be associated with long-face morphology, and strong muscles with a more square-faced appearance. If the activity of the elevator muscles decreases due to lower chewing demands, tooth loss or ongoing pain, bite force declines and the elevator muscles may become hypotrophic, with visible hollowing of temples and cheeks. In contrast, excessive use, such as with ongoing nocturnal bruxism, leads to hypertrophy.

Functional anatomy

Anatomical details of jaw muscles are found in anatomical texts but aspects of jaw function will be briefly discussed; see Chapter 2 for details of jaw muscle physiology.

Closing or elevating the mandible is primarily due to bilateral, symmetrical activity of the masseter, temporalis and medial pterygoid muscles, but during chewing the activity of the masseter muscle is asymmetric, with greater activity on the chewing side. The effect of gravity on the jaw is counteracted by the positive tone of the temporalis muscle, which is considered to be a significant positioner of the jaw. Forceful contraction and tooth contact also involve the masseter and the medial pterygoid muscle. Jaw opening or depression is accomplished by the suprahyoid muscles (anterior digastric, geniohyoid and mylohyoid) with assistance from both lateral pterygoid muscles. The suprahyoid muscles attach the mandible to the hyoid bone. When the hyoid bone is fixed by the action of the infrahyoid muscles, the suprahyoid muscles can participate in the lowering of the mandible. Symmetrical protrusion of the jaw is achieved by bilateral action of the lateral pterygoid muscles. The posterior temporalis and the suprahyoid muscles support mandibular retrusion, with assistance from the deep masseter muscles. Moving the mandible to one side (laterotrusion) involves contraction of the lateral pterygoid muscles on the opposite (contralateral) side from the excursion, assisted by the posterior temporalis muscle in the same side (ipsilateral). However, laterotrusion is usually performed in combination with protrusion of the contralateral side, producing anterolateral jaw movement.

JAW MUSCLE PAIN

Typical symptoms of jaw muscle disorders

Muscle pain is the most common complaint in patients with jaw muscle disorders and the intensity is generally moderate. Muscle pain is diffuse; it may be located to the source of pain, but may also be referred to other structures. Pain from the temporalis muscle is usually felt as headache in the temple and forehead, from the masseter muscle in the jaw and posterior teeth, from the medial pterygoid muscle deep in the cheek and in front of the ear, and from the lateral pterygoid muscle in the zygomatic area. Muscle pain is described as a continuous 'deep dull ache' or 'tightness' or 'pressure', unpleasant and often exhausting, and it is only rarely associated with a general feeling of illness or with other concomitant symptoms. The pain normally has a gradual onset, and it may vary from a feeling of tiredness to a sharper, more severe pain. It may be constant or occur both spontaneously with the jaw at rest, and in response to chewing, stretching, contraction or palpation. Besides pain, a feeling of weakness, stiffness, rigidity or swelling, and a restriction of jaw opening also often characterise jaw muscle disorders.

Muscle pain and pathophysiology

Muscle pain is a form of deep somatic pain capable of causing central excitatory effects. Deep pain inputs also tend to provoke referred pain, hyperalgesia, autonomic effects and secondary muscle co-contraction, as well as emotional reactions. The information leading to the experience of jaw muscle pain is transmitted by free nerve endings, that is, nociceptors (acting as pain receptors), located in muscle, fascia and muscle–tendon complex. Nociceptors relay to the trigeminal subnucleus caudalis and motor nucleus by small diameter and slowly conducting primary trigeminal afferents. Local reflexes elicit motor responses. Ascending pathways to the sensorimotor cortex are the basis of nociceptive localisation, discrimination and evaluation, while input to the hypothalamus and limbic system provide the autonomic and emotional reactions, all of which constitute the experience of pain.

Muscle pain may result from trauma, overuse in terms of sustained or forceful contraction, stretching, ischaemia or hyperaemia. Nociceptors respond to mechanical and chemical stimuli from mechanical forces and endogenous pain-producing substances. Local conditions such as inflammation increase receptivity, so that stimulation becomes more evident at a lowered activation threshold, even by normally innocuous stimuli, and increased spontaneous activity in nociceptors results in soreness and pain. Such sensitisation processes are most likely peripheral mechanisms for muscle tenderness and hyperalgesia (Graven-Nielsen & Mense 2001). Compression and injury to muscle results in direct activation of nociceptors. This occurs by release of prostaglandins from damaged cell membranes which sensitise nociceptors, and by the release of inflammatory mediators and neuro-peptides such as bradykinin and serotonin (from blood vessels), as well as substance P and calcitonin gene-related peptide (from nerve endings). In ischaemic muscle, the induced decrease in oxygen tension and pH releases bradykinin and prostaglandin, which sensitise muscle nociceptors, so that they respond to the force of con-traction. Different simultaneous stimuli may potentate each other; for example, increased extracellular potassium concentration, which occurs in prolonged muscular work, increases sensitivity to chemical stimulation from hypoxia and to mechanical stimuli, such as increased intramuscular pressure and other effects of muscular contraction.

The convergence of the neurones, processing inputs from muscles, joints, and cutaneous and visceral afferents, is the basis for the poor localisation and poor dis-crimination of muscle pain. It is also the cause of referral of pain to other tissues. In second-order neurones of the subnucleus caudalis, an altered responsiveness or sensitisation may take place after longlasting activity in afferent neurones. A range of ascending and descending modulatory mechanisms influences the transmission in the central pathways. Central sensitisation and modulation are the main causes of the often poor correlation in musculoskeletal disorders between the pain experience and the intensity and the duration of the noxious stimuli; this is also true for chronic tension-type headache. The spread of muscle pain and more generalised pain con-ditions may also be related to central sensitisation, as this phenomenon not only comprises increased excitability of neurones of the subnucleus caudalis but also an expansion of their receptive fields.

HISTORY-TAKING AND EXAMINATION OF JAW MUSCLES

This is required as part of a comprehensive evaluation of jaw muscles, which includes a systematic history, examination (palpation and auscultation) of the TM joints

Table 8.1 Evaluation of jaw muscles
History
• Chief complaint (for example, facial pain and headache, jaw stiffness or reduced mandibular opening, difficulty in chewing)
• General features: Medical problems including medication; social and psychosocial factors
• Local features: Mandibular function – mobility, chewing, parafunction. Muscle pain – localisation, onset, course, characteristics (quality, intensity, variation, provocation and alleviation), concomitant symptoms. Previous examination and treatment
Clinical examination
• Orofacial examination: facial appearance; jaw muscles – jaw mobility, tenderness, consistency and volume

and dental occlusion (Table 8.1). The use of provocation tests described in Chapter 5 might also be considered.

Supplementary tests may also be helpful, for example, diagnostic injections and chewing tests. The basis of a proper diagnosis is a thorough identification of symptoms and signs (see also Ch. 7). The patient's chief complaints should be defined and listed according to their importance to the patient. It should be remembered that jaw muscle disorders often coexist with TM joint disorders, or may be a part of a general medical disorder. If a medical disorder is suspected as the primary cause of symptoms or a significant contributing factor, the patient should be referred for medical consultation.

Anamnesis or history

The history-taking of jaw muscle disorders consists ideally of a consultative written questionnaire and an interview. The questionnaire may be mailed to the patient for completion before the initial appointment. A questionnaire would cover general medical as well as dental problems, presence of head and face pain, location of the pain on diagrams (Figure 8.1), and information about restricted jaw movements. Besides giving information on the history, the questionnaire provides a basis for a better clinician–patient understanding. During the interview for history-taking, possible variations of facial morphology, expressions of pain, involuntary jaw movements and the patient's attitudes should be noted. Topics for the interview are given above, but further details from the

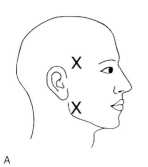
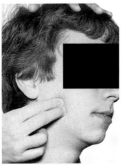

A   B

Fig. 8.1 **A** A patient's indication of the locations of jaw muscle pain in a self-completed written questionnaire. **B** Unilateral palpation of the masseter muscle with a firm pressure by two fingers, rating tenderness according to the verbal and facial expression of the patient.

patient depend on the questioning and the clinician's familiarity with the signs and symptoms of jaw muscle disorders.

As an aid in assessing the intensity of the jaw muscle pain, a 100 mm horizontal VAS (left endpoint 'No pain', right endpoint 'Intolerable pain') may be used, both for the initial interview and for monitoring treatment. The intensity and impact of the pain may also be estimated from:

- medication used
- changes in the patient's social habits
- pain diary listing days with pain.

Clinical examination

The examination has two main purposes:

- to assess jaw function
- to reproduce the patient's pain.

The assessment is achieved primarily by registration of:

- jaw mobility
- pain provocation by maximal jaw opening, by chewing and by muscle palpation.

Jaw function can be assessed routinely by measuring maximum jaw opening in the incisor region, adding the amount of overbite or subtracting the amount of open bite. The reliability of the measures of the vertical range of motion is excellent. Generally, a mandibular opening of less than 40 mm is considered moderately restricted, and less than 30 mm severely restricted. During maximum jaw opening, muscle pain may be provoked or aggravated by stretching the elevator muscles, by the active opening itself, or if the clinician attempts to increase the inter-

incisal distance by putting finger pressure between the upper and lower teeth. A chewing test, for example, gum or cotton rolls, may also be used to provoke or aggravate the pain for diagnostic purposes (Farella et al 2001).

The patient may not easily localise the site of pain, but pain provoked by manual palpation more accurately identifies pain location. Evaluation of tenderness by palpation is normally performed unilaterally with specific pressure by one or two fingers (Fig. 8.1) (Dworkin & LeResche, 1992). The superficial temporalis and masseter muscles are most easily palpated. Palpation of the pterygoid muscles is far more uncertain; a combined extraoral and intraoral approach may be used for the medial pterygoid muscles, and intraoral palpation for the lateral pterygoid muscles.

The response to the palpation may be rated from verbal and reflex responses, for example, as:

- 0 (none – no reflex response)
- 1 (mild – no reflex response)
- 2 (moderate – wincing or grimacing)
- 3 (severe – aversive movement).

A total tenderness score may be calculated from the sum of the ratings of individual muscles. The reliability of manual palpation is generally acceptable for temporalis and masseter muscles only, but the validity has been questioned. Extraoral manual palpation may be supplemented by pressure algometry to increase reliability and validity. The reliability and validity of palpation for localisation of tender points and changes of consistency, such as firm bands, are probably dubious.

Additional assessments to assist diagnosis include:

- provocation tests, described in Chapter 5
- muscle injections with local anaesthetic to confirm the location of the pain.

CLASSIFICATION OF JAW MUSCLE DISORDERS

On the basis of the duration, muscle pain is described as acute or chronic (Table 8.2). Chronic pain is generally recognised as pain that persists beyond the normal healing time. The International Association for the Study of Pain (IASP) recognises 3 months as a convenient separation of acute and chronic pain. Classifications of jaw muscle disorders and associated pain-based signs and symptoms have been described by Dworkin and LeResche (1992) – Research Diagnostic Criteria for Temporomandibular Disorders, Axis I; by Okeson (1996), for the American Academy of Orofacial Pain; and by Fricton and Schiffman (2001).

Table 8.2   Jaw muscle disorders

Myalgic disorders
• Acute
  – Local muscle soreness (postexercise myalgia)
  – Myositis
• Chronic
  – Myofascial pain
  – Tension-type headache
  – Generalised myalgia (for example, fibromyalgia and myalgia associated with systematic diseases)
 	
Other chronic disorders
• Muscle contracture
• Hypertrophy
• Disorders associated with myopathies and neurological disorders (for example, oromandibular dystonia and muscle spasms)

Table 8.3   Tension-type headache
At least two of the following pain characteristics: • Pressing or tightening (non-pulsating) quality; mild or moderate intensity (may inhibit but does not prohibit activities); bilateral location; no aggravation by walking on stairs or similar routine physical activity **Both of the following:** • No vomiting • No more than one of the following: nausea; photophobia; phonophobia

Myalgic disorders

The pathophysiology and aetiology of the myalgic jaw muscle disorder subtypes are not easily differentiated clinically, however they may be described as follows:

• Local muscle soreness or postexercise myalgia is believed to arise after significant or acute overuse of jaw muscles. It presents as pain or stiffness and may arise from excessive bruxism, prolonged chewing or other activities that put great demands on the jaw muscles.

• Myositis is defined as painful inflammation of muscle and connective tissue that results from local causes, such as infection or trauma. If myositis persists, the inflammation may progress to fibrous scarring, causing muscle contracture.

• Myofascial pain is the most common local chronic myalgic disorder of the jaw muscles. Myofascial pain may also be secondary to disc displacements, osteoarthritis and rheumatoid arthritis of the TM joint. It is characterised by local pain associated with specific sites of local tenderness and spread of the pain on palpation. There may be limitation in the range of jaw movement, muscle fatigue and stiffness.

• Tension-type headache associated with disorders of pericranial muscles is chronic localised myalgia in terms of myofascial pain, affecting jaw muscles, especially the temporalis muscles (Table 8.3) (Headache Classification Committee of the International Headache Society 1988). The diagnostic criteria for episodic tension-type headache define this as headache fulfilling the criteria (see Table 8.3) with at least 10 previous headache episodes lasting from 30 minutes to 7 days, but with less than 15 days with headache per month (IHS 2.1.1). Chronic tension-type headache is defined as headache

present for at least 15 days per month for at least 6 months (IHS 2.2.2).

• Chronic generalised myalgia in terms of fibromyalgia may also affect the jaw muscles. Fibromyalgia includes widespread, chronic pain, tiredness and stiffness and bilateral symmetrical tenderness corresponding to at least 11 of 18 particular muscle sites, as well as sleep disturbances and depression.

Other chronic disorders

• The chronic jaw muscle disorder termed 'muscle contracture' that is characterised by fibrositis and limited range of motion is thought to develop from previous trauma.

• Jaw muscle 'hypertrophy', characterised by increased strength and volume, arises from prolonged bruxism or other repetitive forceful activities. These conditions are usually not painful.

• Myopathies or neurological disorders affecting the jaw muscles are seldom associated with muscle pain; genetic and acquired myopathies such as muscle dystrophy, myotonia, polymyositis and dermatomyositis are rather characterised by weakness, atrophy and difficulty in chewing. Neurological disorders affecting jaw muscles hamper oral function, and include oromandibular dystonia with spasmodic episodes of jaw movements, and cerebral palsy with possible daytime bruxism.

TREATMENT OF JAW MUSCLE PAIN AND DISORDERS

The treatment of jaw muscle disorders is designed to reduce pain and improve jaw function. Ideally, the treatment of jaw muscle disorders should be cost-effective and evidence-based. Where evidence is lacking, treatment should be based on well-established accepted clinical practice (Kuttila et al 1998, Pullinger & Seligman 2000). As there is no evidence that local myalgic disorders of jaw muscles are progressive in nature, treatment should also be based on reversible and least-invasive therapies. Such procedures are intended to facilitate the natural healing capacity of the musculoskeletal system, and to involve the patient in the management of the disorder. Regional and widespread disorders, as well as suspicion of general medical conditions, need collaboration with primary care physicians and other medical specialists.

Depending on the type and severity of the jaw muscle disorders, a combination of several treatments may be applied:

- The first step is always counselling, often carried out together with medication for alleviation of pain.
- Analgesics and NSAIDs are normally used for treatment for musculoskeletal pain. NSAIDs (ibuprofen) have been shown to have a positive effect on ischaemic muscle pain. In postexercise jaw muscle soreness, topical NSAID gel is more effective than systemic NSAIDs.
- Muscle relaxants may be used, and 1 month of treatment with diazepam has been shown to reduce chronic jaw muscle myalgia.
- Tricyclic antidepressants may also have a role in the treatment of chronic myofascial pain from jaw muscles. Amitriptyline has a positive effect on chronic tension-type headache, but common side-effects include dry mouth, sedation and constipation.
- Physical therapy is often used as treatment of jaw muscle pain in association with TMDs. Symptoms of TMDs and other chronic musculoskeletal pain improve during treatment with most forms of physical therapy (Feine & Lund 1997). However, most of the therapies have not been proven to be more effective than placebo. These data support the view that it may be the care of the patient itself that matters. Passive exercise and stretching are likely to increase the range of jaw motion but the effect on muscle pain is weak, and there is evidence from the treatment of other musculoskeletal disorders that active exercise of the specific painful area strengthens the muscles, improves function, and reduces pain (Feine & Lund 1997).
- Acupuncture may have a role in treatment of the jaw muscles. There is little evidence for the use of thermal agents, electrical stimulation (TENS), ultrasound, and low-intensity laser therapy for chronic muscle pain and disorders.
- Intraoral appliances such as occlusal stabilisation splints (in hard acrylic resin) have previously been the main treatment for TMDs. However, there is controversy regarding their mode of action. The use of stabilisation splints is supported for localised masticatory myalgia

and TMDs, but their effects are partly due to placebo (Forssell et al 1999).

- Occlusal factors may contribute to TMDs, but only to a minor extent. Occlusal adjustment or prosthetic reconstructions as the treatment for jaw muscle disorders are not recommended.

References

Dworkin S F, LeResche L 1992 Research diagnostic criteria for temporomandibular disorders. Journal of Craniomandibular Disorders: Facial and Oral Pain 6:301–355

Eriksson P O, Haggman-Henrikson B, Nordh E, Zafar H 2000 Co-ordinated mandibular and head–neck movements during rhythmic jaw activities in man. Journal of Dental Research 79:1378–1384

Farella M, Bakke M, Michelotti A, Martina R 2001 Effects of prolonged gum chewing on pain and fatigue in human jaw muscles. European Journal of Oral Sciences 109:81–85

Feine J S, Lund J P 1997 An assessment of the efficacy of physical therapy and physical modalities for the control of chronic musculoskeletal pain (review). Pain 71:5–23

Forssell H, Kalso E, Koskela P et al 1999 Occlusal treatments in temporomandibular disorders: a qualitative systematic review of randomized controlled trials (review). Pain 83:549–560

Fricton J R, Schiffman E 2001 Management of masticatory myalgia and arthralgia. In: Lund J P, Lavigne G J, Dubner R, Sessle B J (eds) Orofacial pain. From basic science to clinical management. The transfer of knowledge in pain research to education. Quintessence, Chicago, pp 235–248

Graven-Nielsen T, Mense S 2001 The peripheral apparatus of muscle pain: evidence from animal and human studies (review). Clinical Journal of Pain 17:2–10

Headache Classification Committee of the International Headache Society 1988. Classification and diagnostic criteria for headache disorders, cranial neuralgias and facial pain. Cephalalgia 8(suppl 7):1–96

Kuttila M, Niemi P M, Kuttila S, Alanen P, Le Bell Y 1998 TMD treatment need in relation to age, gender, stress, and diagnostic subgroup. Journal of Orofacial Pain 12:67–74

Lobbezoo F, Naeije M 2001 Bruxism is mainly regulated centrally, not peripherally. Journal of Oral Rehabilitation 28:1085–1091

Okeson J P (ed) 1996 Differential diagnosis and management considerations of temporomandibular disorders. Orofacial pain: guidelines for assessment, diagnosis and management. The American Academy of Orofacial Pain. Quintessence, Chicago, pp 137–141

Pullinger A G, Seligman D A 2000 Quantification and validation of predictive values of occlusal variables in temporomandibular disorders using a multifactorial analysis. Journal of Prosthetic Dentistry 83:66–75

Further reading

Bakke M 1993 Mandibular elevator muscles: physiology, action, and effect of dental occlusion (review). Scandinavian Journal of Dental Research 101:314–331

Bakke M, Thomsen C E, Vilmann A et al 1996 Ultrasonographic assessment of the swelling of the human masseter muscle after static and dynamic activity. Archives of Oral Biology 41:133–140

Bendtsen L, Jensen R 2000 Amitriptyline reduces myofascial tenderness in patients with chronic tension type headache. Cephalalgia 20:603–610

Dao T T, Lund J P, Lavigne G J 1994 Pain responses to experimental chewing in myofascial pain patients. Journal of Dental Research 73:1163–1167

Drangsholt M, LeResche L 1994 Temporomandibular disorder pain. In: Crombie I K, Croft P R, Linton S J, LeResche L, Von Korff M (eds) Epidemiology of pain. Task force on epidemiology of the International Association for the Study of Pain. IASP Press, Seattle, pp 203–233

Dworkin S F, Huggins K H, LeResche L et al 1990 Epidemiology of signs and symptoms in temporomandibular disorders: clinical signs in cases and controls. Journal of the American Dental Association 120:273–281

Dworkin S F, LeResche L, DeRouen T, von Korff M 1990 Assessing clinical signs of temporomandibular disorders: reliability of clinical examiners. Journal of Prosthetic Dentistry 63:574–579

Kreiner M, Betancor E, Clark G T 2001 Occlusal stabilization appliances. Evidence of their efficacy (review). Journal of the American Dental Association 132:770–777

Layzer R B 1994 Muscle pain, cramps and fatigue. In: Engel A G, Franzini-Amstrong C (eds) Myology. McGraw-Hill, New York, pp 1754–1768

Levine J D 1996 Arthritis and myositis. In: Campbell J N (ed) Pain 1996 – an updated review. IASP Press, Seattle, pp 327–337

Lund J P 2001 Pain and movement. In: Lund J P, Lavigne G J, Dubner R, Sessle B J (eds) Orofacial pain. From basic science to clinical management. The transfer of knowledge in pain research to education. Chicago, Quintessence, pp 151–163

Mense S 1993 Nociception from skeletal muscle in relation to clinical muscle pain (review). Pain 54:241–289

Merskey H, Bogduk N (eds) 1994 Classification of chronic pain, description of chronic pain syndromes and definition of pain terms, 2nd edn. Second task force on taxonomy of the International Association for the Study of Pain. IASP Press, Seattle, pp xi–xiii

Møller E 1966 The chewing apparatus. An electromyographic study of the action of the muscles of mastication and its correlation to facial morphology. Acta Physiologica Scandinavica 69(suppl 280):1–229

National Institutes of Health 1996 Management of temporomandibular disorders. National Institutes of Health Technology Assessment Conference statement. Journal of the American Dental Association 127:1595–1606

Sacchetti G, Lampugnani R, Battistini C, Mandelli V 1980 Response to pathological ischaemic muscle pain to analgesics. British Journal of Clinical Pharmacology 9:165–190

Salmon S 1995.Muscle. In: Williams P L, Bannister L H, Berry M M et al (eds) Gray's anatomy. The anatomical basis of medicine and surgery, 38th edn. Churchill Livingstone, Edinburgh, pp 737–900

Scott J, Huskisson E C 1976 Graphic representation of pain. Pain 2:175–184

Sessle B J 1995 Masticatory muscle disorders: basic science perspectives. In: Sessle B J, Bryant P S, Dionne R A (eds) Temporomandibular disorders and related pain. IASP Press, Seattle, pp 47–61

Singer E, Dionne R 1997 A controlled evaluation of ibuprofen and diazepam for chronic orofacial muscle pain. Journal of Orofacial Pain 11:139–146

Stal P, Eriksson P O, Thornell L E 1996 Differences in capillary supply between human oro-facial, masticatory and limb muscles. Journal of Muscle Research and Cell Motility 17:183–197

Stockstill J, Gross A, McCall W D 1989 Interrater reliability in masticatory muscle palpation. Journal of Craniomandibular Disorders: Facial and Oral Pain 3:143–146

Svensson P, Houe L, Arendt-Nielsen L 1997 Effect of systemic versus topical nonsteroidal antiinflammatory drugs on postexercise jaw-muscle soreness: a placebo-controlled study. Journal of Orofacial Pain 11:353–362

Wolfe F, Smythe H A, Yunus M B et al 1990 The American College of Rheumatology criteria for the classification of fibromyalgia. Report of a multicenter criteria committee. Arthritis and Rheumatism 33:160–172

9 Occlusion and periodontal health

J. De Boever, A. De Boever

Synopsis

Periodontal structures depend on functional occlusal forces to activate the periodontal mechanoreceptors in the neuromuscular physiology of the masticatory system. Occlusal forces stimulate the receptors in the periodontal ligament to regulate jaw movements and the occlusal forces. Without antagonists the periodontal ligament shows some non-functional atrophy. Tooth mobility is the clinical expression of the viscoelastic properties of the ligament and the functional response.

Tooth mobility can change due to general metabolic influences, a traumatic occlusion and inflammation. Premature contacts between the arches can result in trauma to the periodontal structures.

A traumatic occlusion on a healthy periodontium leads to an increased mobility but not to attachment loss. In inflamed periodontal structures traumatic occlusion contributes to a further and faster spread of the inflammation apically and to more bone loss.

A traumatic occlusion, as in a deep bite, may cause stripping of the gingival margins. It is not clear if prematurities or steep occlusal guidance contribute to the occurrence of gingival recession.

On implants, prematurities may result in breakdown of osseointegration. In some cases occlusal corrections will be necessary to eliminate the traumatic influence of a nonphysiological occlusion.

Key points

- Healthy periodontal structures and occlusal forces
- Physiology and clinical aspects of tooth mobility
- Tooth mobility
- Types of occlusal forces
- Trauma from occlusion:
  - Primary trauma in healthy non-inflamed periodontium
  - Primary trauma in healthy but reduced periodontal structures
  - Secondary trauma in the progression of periodontitis
- Implants and occlusal trauma
- Gingival recession and occlusal trauma
- Clinical consequence and procedures

HEALTHY PERIODONTAL STRUCTURES AND OCCLUSAL FORCES

The healthy periodontal structures, including root cementum, periodontal ligament and alveolar bone, form a functional unit or organ. The periodontal ligament is a very specialised interface between tooth and the alveolar bone. It serves as a structural, sensory and nutritive unit supporting the normal oral functions of chewing, swallowing, speaking, etc. It has a very dense network of interconnecting fibres attached to the bone. The supra-crestal fibres are especially important because they maintain the relative position of the teeth in the arch. The collagen fibres in the periodontal ligament are very dense and represent up to 75% of the volume. These so-called 'Sharpey fibres' are apically oriented and embedded both in the alveolar bone and the root cement. The natural dentition has been compared, because of these interconnecting supracrestal fibres, to beads on a string. Teeth function together but have their individual mobility in the alveolus. The entire periodontal ligament has viscoelastic characteristics. The ligament provides tooth fixation, and also force absorption. The thickness of the periodontal ligament is directly related to the forces exerted on it.

The periodontal ligament has a rich and dense vascular and nervous network. The ligament contains proprioceptors for movement and positioning and mechanoreceptors for touch, pain and pressure. They regulate muscle function and occlusal forces to avoid overload and damage of the teeth and the alveolar bone. The periodontal ligament distributes and absorbs forces. Under physiological conditions the occlusal forces are transferred to alveolar bone and further to the mandible, the maxilla and the entire skull. The alveolar process has a pronounced capacity for modelling and remodelling under functional loading. The alveolar process remodels at a rate of 20% per year. The basal bone does not have this capacity. The periodontal ligament and alveolar bone need the functional stimulus of the occlusion to maintain their physiological, healthy condition.

TOOTH MOBILITY

Physiological tooth mobility is the result of the histological characteristics of the periodontal ligament. Physiological tooth mobility, in the horizontal as well as in the vertical direction, is different between single root and multirooted teeth and is determined by the width, height and quality of the periodontal ligament (Fig. 9.1).

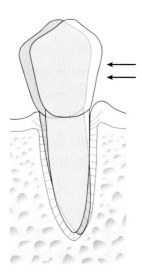

Fig. 9.1 Physiological tooth mobility in a healthy periodontium is determined by the bone height, the form of the root and the magnitude of the applied force, and the extent is limited.

In the vertical direction, the displacement is 0.02 mm by small forces up to 1 N. Under larger vertical forces, the tooth is moved in an apical direction because venous fluid and blood of the periodontal structures is pushed towards the venous lacunae and the cancellous bone. It takes 1–2 minutes before the tooth returns to its normal position after releasing an applied occlusal force. This explains the fact that tooth mobility is decreased after chewing, and the tooth is then in a more apical position.

In healthy conditions, the teeth move in a horizontal plane, under a force of 500 g, as follows (Mühlemann 1960):

- incisors: 0.1–0.12 mm
- canines: 0.05–0.09 mm
- premolars: 0.08–0.1 mm
- molars: 0.04–0.08 mm.

Tooth mobility can also be estimated using the Periotest (Siemens AG, Germany), an electronic device that measures the reaction of the periodontium to a defined percussion force.

Under higher occlusal loads, the forces are transmitted to the bone, with slight deformation of the alveolar process as a result. The force is also transmitted to neighbouring teeth through the interproximal contacts.

Evaluation of tooth mobility

The exact measurement of individual tooth mobility (periodontometry) is necessary for research purposes. Clinically, an estimation of tooth mobility is performed by loading the tooth in an anterolateral direction with two instruments.

Four possible grades of tooth mobility are considered:

- grade 0: physiological mobility
- grade 1: increased mobility but less than 1 mm in total
- grade 2: pronounced increase; more than 1 mm in total
- grade 3: more than 1 mm displacement combined with a displacement in vertical direction (tooth can be intruded).

Increased mobility can also be observed on radiographs: there is a widening of the periodontal space without vertical or angular bone resorption and without increased probing depth of the periodontal pocket (Figs 9.2 and 9.3).

Aetiological factors of hyper- and hypomobility

Excessive occlusal forces or premature contacts on teeth are the primary aetiologic factors for hypermobility.

There is an increased mobility during pregnancy because of the increase in the fluid content of the periodontal structures, an increased vascularity and a proliferation of

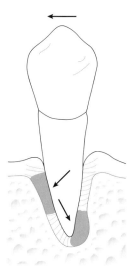

Fig. 9.2 Forces applied in one direction on the tooth give a widening of the periodontal ligament at the bone margin at the other side and in the apical area on the same side of the force.

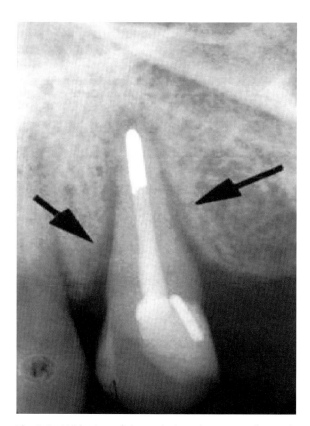

Fig. 9.3 Widening of the periodontal space as observed on radiographs.

capillaries into the periodontal tissues. Systemic diseases such as non-Hodgkin's lymphoma, scleroderma and Cushing's syndrome may lead to increased mobility. Hypermobility may be observed in cases of severe periodontal inflammation (periodontitis), teeth with a healthy but reduced periodontal support (that is, in patients after successful periodontal treatment), or in the first weeks after periodontal surgery.

Normal physiological mobility is decreased in the elderly and in the absence of antagonist teeth. In cases of severe bruxism and clenching the mobility decreases ('ankylosing effect'). Without antagonists and therefore without functional stimulation, teeth will either overerupt or become ankylosed. The periodontal ligament becomes thinner and non-functional.

Evaluation of the changes in occlusal mobility can be helpful in the diagnosis of occlusal dysfunction, parafunction and in the evaluation of occlusal treatment procedures.

TYPES OF OCCLUSAL FORCES

The reaction of the bone and ligament depends on the magnitude, duration and direction of the forces. Different types of occlusal forces can be recognised:

- *Physiologically normal occlusal forces in chewing and swallowing*: small and rarely exceeding 5 N. They provide the positive stimulus to maintaining the periodontium and the alveolar bone in a healthy and functional condition.
- *Impact forces*: mainly high but of short duration. The periodontium can sustain high forces during a short period; however, forces exceeding the viscoelastic buffer capacities of the periodontal ligament will result in fracture of tooth and bone.
- *Continuous forces*: very low forces (for example, orthodontic forces), but continuously applied in one direction are effective in displacing a tooth by remodelling the alveolus.
- *Jiggling forces*: intermittent forces in two different directions (premature contacts on, for example, crowns, fillings) result in widening of the alveolus and in increased mobility.

TRAUMA FROM OCCLUSION

Trauma from occlusion has been defined as structural and functional changes in the periodontal tissues caused by excessive occlusal forces. Some of these changes are adaptive, while others should be considered pathological. Occlusal trauma can be acute if caused by external impact

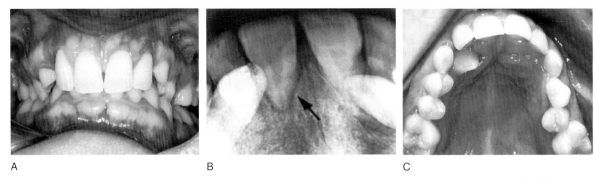

A   B   C

Fig. 9.4 Clinical example of a primary occlusal trauma in a young girl with a deep bite and a persistent deciduous canine. **A** Frontal view showing the deep bite. **B** Palatal view, with the primary trauma on the palatal mucosa caused by the lower canine. When the patient closes, the lower canine is forced in between the upper canine and the central and lateral incisors. **C** This traumatic occlusion causes the widening of the periodontal space, as seen on the radiograph.

forces or chronic if caused by internal occlusal factors (premature contacts, grinding). Chronic occlusal trauma can be understood as primary and secondary trauma.

Occlusal trauma is the overall process by which *traumatic occlusion* (that is, an occlusion that produces forces that cause injury) produces injury to the attachment apparatus.

Primary occlusal trauma

Primary occlusal trauma is caused by excessive and non-physiological forces exerted on teeth with a normal, healthy and non-inflamed periodontium. The forces may be exerted on the periodontal structures in one direction (orthodontic forces) or as 'jiggling' forces.

Forces in one direction: orthodontic forces

Forces in one direction cause tipping of the tooth in the opposite direction or tooth displacement parallel to the force resulting in a 'bodily movement'.

In the periodontal ligament, zones of compression and zones of tension are found, inducing increased resorption. The clinical result is a (temporary) increased mobility. However, there are no changes in the supracrestal fibres, no loss of periodontal attachment, or an increased probing pocket depth. The increased tooth mobility is functional adaptation to the forces exerted on that tooth. If the forces are too high and above the adaptation level, an aseptic necrosis in the tension zone of the periodontal ligament occurs, characterised by hyalinisation. In the compression zone, pressure stimulates osteoclasts in the adjacent bone and the alveolar wall is resorbed until a new connection is formed with the hyalinised bone ('undermining resorption'). In the tension zone, bone apposition and rupture of the collagen fibres occur. After removal of the force the periodontal ligament is reorganised and after some time

develops a normal histological appearance. If the applied forces are too high, root resorption occurs in the middle of the hyalinised tissues. This resorption continues for a variable time, resulting in shorter roots, frequently seen after orthodontic treatment.

Jiggling forces

Jiggling forces, coming from different and opposite directions, cause more complex histological changes in the ligament. Theoretically the same events (hyalinisation, resorption) occur, however, they are not clearly separated.

There are no distinct zones of pressure and tension. Histologically, there is apposition and resorption on either side of the periodontal ligament, resulting in a widening of the periodontal space (Fig. 9.4). This may be observed on radiographs. This phenomenon explains the increased mobility without pocket formation, migration and tipping.

The clinical phenomena are not only dependent on the magnitude of the forces, but also on the crown–root relationship, the position in the arch, the direction of the long axis, and the pressure of tongue and cheek musculature (Fig. 9.5). The interarch relationship (for example, deep bite) influences the extent of the trauma caused by jiggling forces. The hypermobility is found as long as the forces are exerted on the tooth: there is no adaptation. Hypermobility is therefore not a sign of an ongoing process, but may be the result of a previous jiggling force.

The long-term prognosis of teeth with increased mobility is poor, and is a complicating factor if they are used as abutment in prosthodontic reconstruction.

Successful periodontal treatment leads to healthy but reduced periodontal structures. Jiggling forces exerted on the teeth in this condition result in a pronounced increase in tooth mobility because the point of rotation (fulcrum) is closer to the apex than normal. This is uncomfortable for

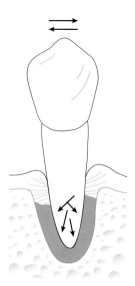

Fig. 9.5 Under jiggling forces in a healthy periodontium, the periodontal ligament space is widened, resulting in more tooth mobility but not in marginal bone resorption or attachment loss.

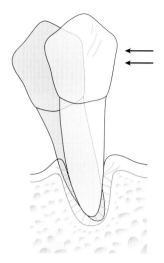

Fig. 9.6 In cases of a healthy but reduced periodontium the tooth mobility (measured at the crown level) is increased for the same force, as compared with a tooth with a complete periodontium, because of the more apical position of the fulcrum.

the patient and might be an indication for splinting of teeth (Fig. 9.6).

Secondary occlusal trauma

Secondary trauma from occlusion is defined as the trauma caused by excessive and premature occlusal forces on teeth with an inflamed periodontium. A number of animal experiments and clinical epidemiological studies investigated the role of occlusion in the pathogenesis of periodontitis. In his original studies in the 1960s, Glickman (Glickman & Smulow 1967) formulated the hypothesis that premature contacts and excessive occlusal forces could be a co-factor in the progression of periodontal disease by changing the pathway and spread of inflammation into the deeper periodontal tissues. Glickman hypothesised that the gingival zone was a *'zone for irritation'* by the microbial plaque; the supracrestal fibres were then considered to be a *'zone of co-destruction'* under the influence of a faulty occlusion (Fig. 9.7).

Clinically, vertical bone resorption and the formation of infrabony defects should be an indication for occlusal trauma.

Animal experiments

Animal experiments investigating the influence of a faulty occlusion on the progression of periodontal disease were published by Swedish investigators between 1970

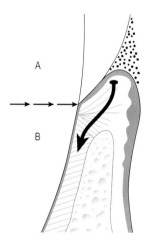

Fig. 9.7 Role of traumatic occlusion in the progression of periodontitis according to Glickman & Smulow (1967). In the presence of microbial plaque and inflammation, **A** is the 'zone of irritation' and **B** the 'zone of co-destruction' where the prematurities are co-destructive by changing the inflammatory pathway.

and 1980 using the beagle dog model, and by American investigators using the squirrel monkey model. In spite of the many remaining questions and controversies, few animal studies have been published since then.

From these studies the following conclusions may be drawn:

- In the absence of marginal inflammation, jiggling forces do not induce more bone resorption nor a shift of the epithelial attachment in an apical direction.
- In the case of marginal inflammation (gingivitis), occlusal overload has no influence.
- Jiggling forces on teeth with periodontal disease result in more bone loss and more loss of connective tissue attachment (Ericsson & Lindhe 1982).
- Jiggling forces induce a faster shift of microbial plaque in the apical direction in the pocket (Fig. 9.8).
- One single trauma does not influence the pathogenesis; the forces have to be chronic.
- Treatment of periodontal inflammation without elimination of the premature contacts results in decreased tooth mobility, an increase in bone density, but no change of bone level.
- After periodontal treatment with scaling and root-planing, the presence or absence of prematurities have no influence on the microbial repopulation of the deepened pockets.

It must be mentioned that some animal studies did not reach the same definitive conclusions, due to differences in experimental setup and different animal models. The results of experimental animal studies cannot therefore be directly extrapolated to the human situation.

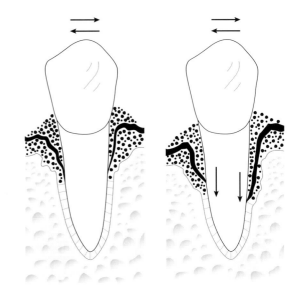

Fig. 9.8 In applying jiggling forces on an inflamed, untreated periodontium with existing infrabony pockets (**A**), the bone destruction is accelerated and the bacteria move more apically (**B**).

Clinical epidemiological studies

Given the complexity of the occlusal and periodontal interaction and the multifactorial aspect of the pathology, very few human studies have been published. Most studies have a limited number of subjects and the results are analysed on a subject basis rather than on a tooth basis. The studies have been recently summarised by Hallmon (Hallmon 1999). A number of cross-sectional epidemiological studies found either no relationship between the presence of premature contacts and increased probing depth or bone loss, while others reported that mobility and radiographic evidence of a widened periodontal ligament were associated with increased pocket depth, attachment loss and bone loss (Jin & Cao 1992). More recent longitudinal studies (Harrel & Nunn 2001) found that teeth with premature contacts at initial examination had a deeper probing pocket depth, an increased mobility and a worse prognosis. At the 1 year examination, teeth without premature contacts originally, or teeth where premature contacts had been removed, showed a 66% reduced chance of a worsening periodontal situation. After a few months, teeth with prematurities showed an increased probing depth compared with the teeth receiving occlusal adjustment. It was concluded that premature contacts are a 'catalyst' in the progression of periodontal disease.

It has also been shown that in the same patient more periodontopathogens are found in pockets around hypermobile teeth, than in teeth with normal mobility. This can lead to the hypothesis that the increased mobility changes the ecosystem in the pocket, favouring growth of these bacteria.

TRAUMA FROM OCCLUSION AND IMPLANTS

Endosseous implants have no periodontal ligament as an intimate implant–alveolar bone contact exists ('functional ankylosis'). Implant failure can occur not only because of bacterial infection (peri-implantitis) but also because of occlusal overload (biomechanical failure) in combination with immunological host factors (Esposito et al 1998).

Occlusal overload results in 'osseodisintegration' over the complete implant surface without clinically detectable pocket formation or signs of inflammation. Often the implant has no increased mobility in spite of pronounced bone resorption along its entire surface. Clinical measurement of implant mobility is not an accurate tool for evaluating osseointegration or disintegration of an implant until late in the pathological process. If increased implant mobility occurs, osseointegration is by then usually destroyed.

GINGIVAL TRAUMA FROM OCCLUSION

Gingival recession may be provoked by direct contact of the teeth with the gingiva, as in severe overbite, where the upper incisors damage the buccal gingiva of the lower incisors. This problem is not easy to solve and may involve orthodontic treatment, orthognathic surgery or extensive prosthetic rehabilitation requiring an increase in vertical dimension.

It has been stated that gingival recession occurs with functional overload and/or premature contacts, as in the buccal surface of upper canines where there is a steep lateral canine guidance. Those cervical surfaces also show enamel abraction. There is still controversy regarding whether or not overload is an aetiological factor in the recession, and consequently whether or not the occlusion and the lateral guidance should be changed.

PRACTICAL CLINICAL CONCLUSIONS AND GUIDELINES

• In a healthy non-inflamed dentition, traumatic occlusion leads to hypermobility of some teeth; if hypermobility, radiological widening of periodontal ligament space or pronounced cervical abraction is found, the occlusion should be analysed and corrected. Simple uncomplicated, non-time-consuming procedures are in most cases adequate to restore a physiological situation and to reduce hypermobility.

• In cases of a healthy but reduced periodontium, increased mobility may also be reduced by occlusal adjustment; it should be recognised that tooth mobility in such cases, based on the mechanical situation, is nevertheless increased. It may be necessary to splint the teeth to increase the functional comfort and to avoid direct fracture. This may include very mobile teeth with a healthy but reduced periodontium, but complicates the clinical procedures.

• In cases of secondary occlusal trauma, treating the inflammation is of primary importance and should be the first step in treatment planning. From the literature it can be concluded that prematurities may play a role in the progression of the periodontitis.

• A simple correction of the occlusion, if necessary, should be included in the initial phase of periodontal treatment. This results in more gain in attachment level during periodontal treatment, and may contribute to better healing of periodontal tissues.

• There are some indications that removing premature tooth contacts improves the prognosis of periodontally involved tissues.

• If some teeth do not react to conventional periodontal treatment as expected, further investigation should not only include periodontal re-examination and microbiological testing, but also more extensive occlusal analysis.

• As implant overload leads to bone resorption without the warning signal of inflammation, deep peri-implantitis pockets or (in the early stage) increased mobility, evaluation of the occlusion and radiographs should be included in regular maintenance programmes.

 ## References

Ericsson I, Lindhe J 1982 The effect of long standing jiggling on the experimental marginal periodontitis in the beagle dog. Journal of Clinical Periodontology 9:495

Esposito M, Hirsch J M, Lekholm U, Thomsen P 1998 Biological factors contributing to failures of osseointegrated implants. II. Etiopathogenesis. European Journal of Oral Sciences 106:721–764

Glickman I, Smulow I B 1967 Further observation on the effects of trauma from occlusion. Journal of Periodontology 38:280

Hallmon W 1999 Occlusal trauma: effect and impact on the periodontium. Annals of Periodontology 4:102

Harrel S K, Nunn M E 2001 The effect of occlusal discrepancies upon periodontitis. II. Relationships of occlusal treatment to the progression of periodontal disease. Journal of Periodontology 72:495–505

Jin L, Cao C 1992 Clinical diagnosis of trauma from occlusion and its relation with severity of periodontitis. Journal of Clinical Periodontology 19:92–97

Mühlemann H R 1960 Ten years of tooth mobility measurements. Journal of Periodontology 31:110–122

 ## Further reading

Beertsen W, McCulloch C A G, Sodek J 1997 The periodontal ligament: a unique, multifunctional connective tissue. Periodontology 2000 13:20–40

Burgett F G, Ramfjord S P, Nissle R R et al 1992 A randomized trial of occlusal adjustment in the treatment of periodontitis. Journal of Clinical Periodontology 19:381–387

Gher M 1996 Non surgical pocket therapy: dental occlusion. Annals of Periodontology 1:567–580

Giargia M, Lindhe J 1997 Tooth mobility and periodontal disease. Journal of Clinical Periodontology 24:785–791

Grant D A, Flynn M J, Slots J 1995 Periodontal microbiota of mobile and non-mobile teeth. Journal of Periodontology 66:386–390

Kaufman H, Carranza F A, Enders B, Neuman M G, Murphy N 1984 Influence of trauma from occlusion on the bacterial re-population of periodontal pockets in dogs. Journal of Periodontology 55:86–92

McCulloch C A G, Kekic P, McKee M D 2000 Role of physical forces in regulating the form and function of the periodontal ligament. Periodontology 24:56–72

Polson A M II 1974 Co-destructive factors of periodontitis and mechanically produced injury. Journal of Periodontal Research 9:108–113

Schulte W, Hoedt B, Lukas D, Maune M, Steppeler M 1992 Periotest for measuring periodontal characteristics. Correlation with periodontal bone loss. Journal of Periodontal Research 27:181–190

Wang H, Burgett F G, Shyt Y, Ramfjord S 1994 The influence of molar furcation involvement and mobility on future clinical periodontal attachment loss. Journal of Periodontology 65:25–29

10 Occlusion and orthodontics

A. Darendeliler, O. Kharbanda

PART 1: CHILDREN AND YOUNG ADULTS

Synopsis

An overview of concepts of normal occlusion and malocclusion is presented from an orthodontic viewpoint. Orthodontists perceive occlusion as tooth alignment and interarch alignment in relation to the underlying skeletal bases and facial soft tissues. Functional and dynamic aspects of occlusion are now also being incorporated into objectives of orthodontic treatment. A classification of malocclusion and its characteristics is presented. Features of postorthodontic optimal occlusion following treatment with fixed appliances are presented.

Key points

- Orthodontics is aimed at providing a well-functioning and anatomically optimal occlusion that is in harmony with the underlying skeletal base, is aesthetically pleasing and functionally stable with age
- Malocclusion is not an organic disease but a deviation from normal, that can have infinite variations
- Malocclusion has aesthetic, functional and superimposed psychological implications
- Development of normal occlusion/ malocclusion is the outcome of complex interactions of jaw growth, growth of the cranium and face, development of the dentition, eruption timing and sequence of eruption, soft-tissue function and maturation. These features are governed by the genetic architecture and yet are greatly influenced by environmental factors, including nutrition, mode of respiration, habits and integrity/maintenance of the deciduous dentition
- Early recognition of malocclusion and its timely interception can minimise or eliminate certain forms of malocclusion
- Growth modification of growing class II malocclusion is now a recognised and accepted modality of treatment
- Growth modification in growing class III malocclusion is relatively less predictable, yet recommended in certain types of maxillary hypoplasia
- Full-banded fixed appliance therapy is the most effective mode of treatment of malocclusions of dental origin and some variations of skeletal malocclusions

OPTIMAL OCCLUSION: PHILOSOPHY OF EVIDENCE FOR ORTHODONTICS

The concept and philosophy of 'normal' occlusion in orthodontics developed in relation to the teeth having a 'specific arrangement' in the dental arches (intra-arch) and in relation to opposing arches (inter-arch). The well-aligned dental arches that have 'normal' labial and buccal overjet, some overbite and have a 'normal' anteroposterior relationship between maxillary and mandibular arches constitute normal occlusion.

Historically, cusp-to-fossa relationships of upper and lower teeth were regarded as being of special significance. In the late nineteenth and early twentieth centuries, Angle emphasised the relationship of the mesiobuccal cusp of the maxillary first molar to the buccal groove of the mandibular first molar as the 'key factor' in the establishment of a class I molar 'normal' relationship. He considered the maxillary first molar to be a stable tooth, which occupied a distinct relationship in the maxillary bone. The position of each dental unit in the arch was also described in terms of its unique 'axial inclination'.

Clinical observations on occlusion were considered both within an arch and in relation to the opposing arches. Within the arch the following were considered: tight proximal contacts, labiolingual/buccolingual placement, rotation and labiolingual/mesiodistal inclination. Angle also believed that a full complement of teeth was essential for teeth to be in balance with facial harmony.

Following Angle, clinical research evidence was considered. Studies from the University of Illinois reported that the maxillary first molar did not always have a distinct relationship with the key ridge in the maxilla. The research by Begg on the occlusion of Australian Aborigines suggested that reduction in tooth substance by proximal and occlusal wear was physiological (Begg 1954). Tweed considered the face and the occlusion from the perspective of axial inclination of the lower incisors and their relationship with the mandibular plane as a guide for determining normal/abnormal relationships of other dental units to their basal bones. His cephalometric studies provided evidence that in order to achieve a balance of lower incisors with basal bone it may be necessary to extract some teeth (Tweed 1946).

The advent of cephalometrics and studies on 'facial variations' reconfirmed many of the earlier empirical clinical observations that normal occlusion may exist in harmony with skeletal bases only if the skeletal bases and facial bones follow normal growth and development. Cephalometric studies provided an understanding of how the dentition and the occlusion and underlying skeletal structures grow over time, and differentiated normal and abnormal growing faces and occlusion.

In 1972, Andrews' analysis of dental casts of normal (non-orthodontic normal occlusion/no history of orthodontic treatment) subjects generated a database of occlusal characteristics that have been grouped into 'six keys of occlusion':

1. Molar relationships. In addition to the previously described features of the mesiobuccal and mesiolingual cusps of the maxillary first molar with the mandibular first molar, Andrews added that the distal surface of the distobuccal cusp of the maxillary first molar occluded with the mesial surface of the mesiobuccal cusp of the mandibular second molar.
2. Crown angulations (mesiodistal tip). Andrews reconfirmed the axial inclination of the teeth and termed it 'tip'. The crown tip is expressed in degrees and is variable for each tooth.
3. Crown inclination (labiolingual or buccolingual). Each tooth crown in the arch has a distinct bucco/labiolingual inclination, designated as 'torque', which is distinct for each tooth crown.
4. Rotations. In optimal occlusion, there should be no tooth rotation. A rotated molar occupies more space in the arch and does not allow optimal occlusion.
5. All teeth in the arch should have tight proximal contact.
6. Flat or mild curve of Spee is a prerequisite of normal occlusion. A deep curve of Spee is suggestive of malocclusion.

The 'six keys' are meaningful for normal occlusion (Fig. 10.1), not because they are consistently seen in all cases but because the 'lack of even one' may suggest incomplete orthodontic treatment. Orthodontic treatment goals should aim to attain Andrews' six keys. Andrews' proposals on tip and torque values have been incorporated into orthodontic brackets and tubes of fixed appliances. Such appliances are generically called 'pre-adjusted' because they facilitate tooth movement in optimal inclinations and angulations without requiring many adjustments.

Tip and torque values suggested by Andrews are supposedly more suitable for Caucasians. There are variations in Asians, African-Americans and other races, but they follow similar features.

Roth (1981) suggested that orthodontic treatment goals should also include intercuspal contact position (ICP) or centric occlusion coincident with retruded contact position (RCP) or centric relation. In protrusive excursions, eight lower anterior teeth should ideally contact six upper anterior teeth and provide smooth lateral and anterior guidance.

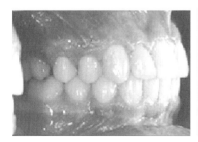 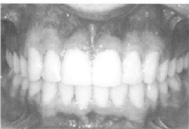 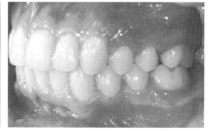

Fig. 10.1 Normal occlusion: occlusion following non-extraction orthodontic treatment.

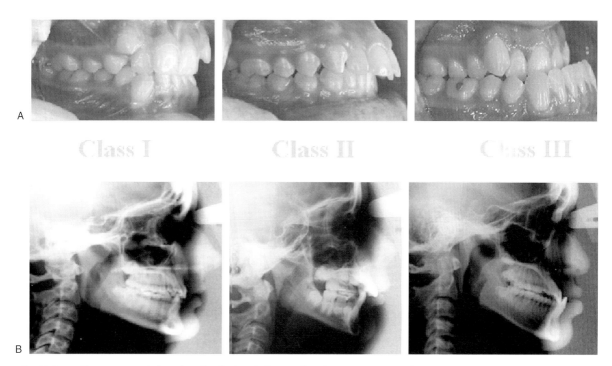

Fig. 10.2   A Three types of dental malocclusion: left to right, class I, II and III. **B** Three types of skeletal malocclusion: left to right, classes I, II and III.

MALOCCLUSION

Any significant deviation from normal occlusion may be termed 'malocclusion'. Current orthodontic understanding of occlusion necessitates that teeth should have normal intra- and interarch relationships, be in harmony with the underlying skeletal bases, and exhibit a well-balanced face. In addition, deviations in normal functional relationships suggest malocclusion.

Malocclusion may be of dental or skeletal origin, or both. Deviations could occur in all the dimensions, that is, anteroposterior, vertical or transverse, in isolation or in combinations of varying severity.

Deviations range from minor, such as slight alterations in arch position, tooth tip or tooth rotation, to more severe forms of crowding, spacing or abnormal overjet and overbite and their combinations of varying severity. Minor malocclusions may have insignificant functional consequences, yet may generate psychosocial concerns for child or adult. While more severe malocclusion in other individuals may or may not be of any concern, it may be associated with functional problems.

Classification of malocclusion

In order to standardise description and treatment planning, malocclusion based on molar relationships was grouped into three classes (Angle 1906), using Roman numerals (I, II, III) to denote the classes and Arabic numerals (1, 2) to denote divisions. A malocclusion that exists unilaterally is termed a subdivision. Using the maxillary first molar as a reference, the classification is: normal mesiodistal (anteroposterior) relationship of the upper and lower first molars (class I); and variations, that is, a distal lower arch (class II), or mesial lower arch (class III) relationship. Figure 10.2A illustrates dental classes I, II and III.

• *Class I malocclusion* exists when maxillary and mandibular first molar teeth have a normal cusp-to-fossa relationship, but there may be deviations in the arrangement of teeth, intra-arch, interarch or both. The common features of class I malocclusions include:
• maxillary protrusion
• crowding/spacing
• anterior/posterior crossbites

- deep/open bite
- midline shift
- combinations of the above.

• *Class II malocclusion* (also called distal occlusion) – the lower first molar is distal to its normal relationship with the maxillary first molar; the mesiobuccal cusp of the maxillary first molar falls mesial to the buccal groove of the mandibular first molar. The usual features of such malocclusions are:

- distal positioning of lower canines (class II canine)
- maxillary protrusion
- deep bite
- inter- and/or intra-arch deviations in teeth.

Class II malocclusions associated with proclined maxillary incisors are called *division 1* or with retroclined maxillary incisors *division 2*.

• *Class III malocclusion* exists when the lower arch (mandibular first molar) is mesial to its normal relationship with the maxillary first molar, that is, the mesiobuccal cusp of the maxillary first molar falls distal to the buccal groove of the lower first molar.

The advent of cephalometrics allowed study of the morphology of the cranium, face and jaws, which provided a better understanding of the skeletal and dental components of malocclusion. This allowed classification of skeletal jaw relationships. Figure 10.2B describes three types of skeletal malocclusion.

• *Skeletal class I: Orthognathic or normal* – maxillary and mandibular skeletal bases are in a normal anteroposterior relationship. Skeletal class I jaw relationship does not necessitate a dental class I relationship. A dental class II or class III malocclusion may occur on a skeletal class I base.

• *Skeletal class II: Distal jaw relationship* exhibits an anteroposterior discrepancy between the maxillary and mandibular bases. A skeletal class II relationship could arise from a smaller (or posteriorly positioned) mandible or an anteriorly placed (or larger) maxilla, or a combination of both. A class I or class II dental mal-occlusion may be observed on skeletal class II bases, but a dental class III relationship on a skeletal class II base is extremely unusual.

• *Skeletal Class III: Mesial jaw relationship* exists when the mandibular skeletal base is mesial to the maxillary base in an anteroposterior relationship. Such a relation-ship could arise when there is a normal maxilla and a large mandible or as a pseudo-class III with a small maxilla and a normal-sized mandible. A varying combination of maxillary deficiency and mandibular prognathism also occurs. Depending upon the severity and location of the skeletal class III dysplasia, a class I or class III dental relationship might exist.

OCCLUSION FOLLOWING ORTHODONTIC TREATMENT

Non-extraction era

The development of a more scientific approach from the beginning of the twentieth century was mainly devoted to refinement of 'appliance(s)', which could effectively move teeth into the preconceived concept of 'normal dental relationship'. The treatment by expansion and alignment could provide normal alignment and cusp-to-fossa relationships, but was not always in harmony with the underlying skeletal bases and facial soft tissues.

Extraction era: search for the evidence

Tweed (1945) reviewed his treated cases that (1) did not result in good facial aesthetics; (2) had relapsed; (3) showed facial balance and a stable occlusion. Clinical observations were supported by cephalometric studies; in subjects with a balanced face and good occlusion (orthodontically treated), mandibular incisors were close to 90° to the mandibular plane (IMPA) and their Frankfort mandibular plane angle (FMA) was about 25°. Accordingly, the maxillary arch required alignment to normal overjet with the mandibular incisors. To upright mandibular incisors (bringing close to 90°), space was required in the arch, which could be obtained with extracting first premolars. Tweed's extraction approach was further supported by Begg, who reported that proximal reduction of tooth surfaces was an essential part of physiological occlusion (Begg 1954). Similarly, maxillary expansion may be insufficient in the correction of large overjet/crowding, and alignment and extraction of some teeth may be unavoidable.

This resulted in extractions being performed without the necessary consideration of the remaining growth in children and their effect on the adult facial profile. The long-term growth studies which are now available need to be considered in orthodontic treatment planning, together with specific racial and ethnic characteristics, which show variations in cephalometric parameters. It has since been realised that extractions should be used with caution following a comprehensive assessment that includes space requirements, growth trend or anticipated growth, soft-tissue profile and treatment mechanics.

Occlusion without extraction

The occlusal relationships following non-extraction orthodontic treatment are similar to that of an occlusion with a full complement of teeth (Fig. 10.3).

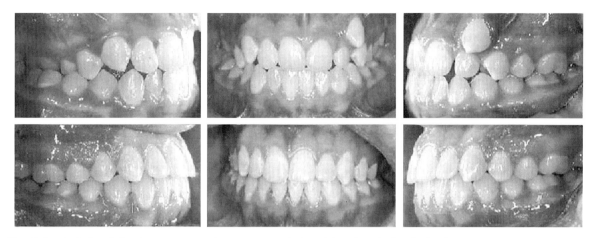

Fig. 10.3 Occlusion following non-extraction treatment: before (above) and after (below) treatment.

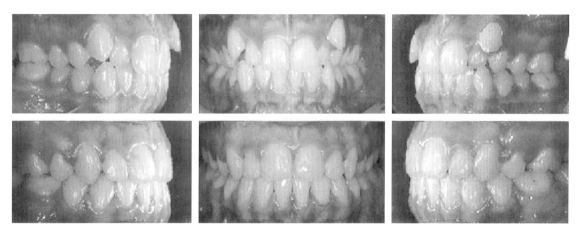

Fig. 10.4 Occlusion following extraction of four premolars: before (above) and after (below) treatment.

Occlusion with extraction

Four first premolars

Class I malocclusion The extraction space achieved following premolar extraction in both arches is utilised for arch alignment and establishment of optimal overjet and overbite. With the use of preadjusted appliances, normal mesiodistal angulation (tip) and labiolingual inclinations (torque) of the teeth may be achieved. However, in some cases proximal contact of the distal surface of the canine with that of the mesial surface of the second premolars will be less than ideal, due to the smaller convexity of the mesial surface of the second premolar. The maxillary second premolars are usually smaller than the first premolars.

Class II malocclusion The extraction space in the maxillary arch is used to correct overjet and crowding. The extraction space in the lower arch is used to reduce the curve of Spee, crowding and mesial movement

of lower molars, to achieve class I molar relationship (Fig. 10.4).

Maxillary first premolars and mandibular second premolars

Lower second premolar extractions provide greater mesial movement of the lower first molars for the correction of class II to class I molar relationships where space requirements in the lower anterior segment are small. This approach is common in treatment of class II division 1 dental malocclusion.

Maxillary first premolars only: therapeutic class II occlusion

In certain forms of class II malocclusion, where the lower arch is well aligned, protrusion may be corrected by extraction of first premolars in the upper arch only. The

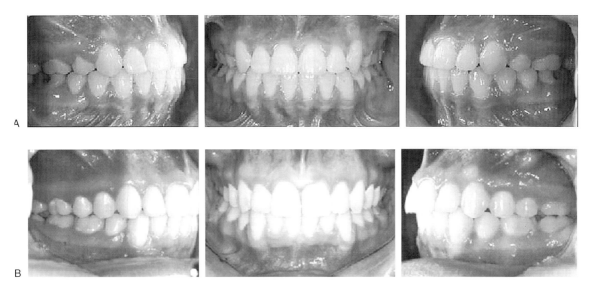

Fig. 10.5 **A** Therapeutic class II. **B** Therapeutic class III.

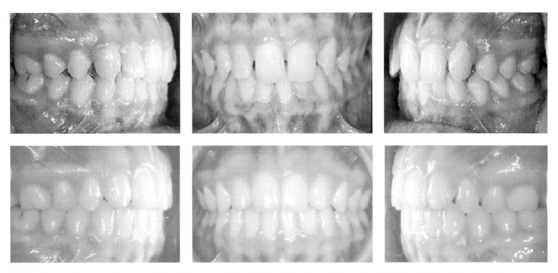

Fig. 10.6 Case of space closure with missing maxillary laterals before (above) and after (below) treatment.

postorthodontic occlusion would have a normal overjet and overbite, with maxillary second premolars and molars in a full cusp class II relationship with the mandibular arch. Under these conditions the mesiobuccal cusp of the maxillary first molar articulates in the embrasure between the mandibular first molar and second premolar. The distobuccal cusp of the maxillary molar articulates with the mandibular first molar mesiobuccal groove (Fig. 10.5A).

Mandibular first premolars: therapeutic class III occlusion

In certain forms of class III malocclusion, treatment might involve alignment of the maxillary arch, proclination of the upper anteriors and retraction of the mandibular incisors, while the molars are maintained in a class III malocclusion. The space for retraction and retroclination of the lower incisors may need to be obtained by extraction of lower first or second premolars. Post-orthodontic occlusion will have a class III molar and premolar relation and class I canine relation with normal overjet and overbite (Fig. 10.5B).

Occlusion with missing maxillary laterals

Orthodontic treatment with missing maxillary laterals may include regaining space and restoration of laterals. In other situations where extraction space may be required for the correction of the malocclusion, the lateral incisor space can be closed by moving the maxillary canines mesially. Postorthodontic (normal) occlusion in such a

case would substitute the first premolars for the maxillary canines and the canines for the laterals. Canines need to be modified for aesthetics and would require reshaping of the labial surface, cusp tip and proximal surfaces, to more closely resemble the laterals. The mesial and distal slopes may be modified with composite resin. The functional anterior guidance would necessitate some adjustment of the lingual surface. The maxillary first premolar may substitute for the maxillary canine, and the intra-arch 'canine' relationship has the mesial slope of the maxillary first premolar with the distal of the lower canine. The maxillary first premolar may need reshaping of the mesiobuccal slope and some reduction of the lingual cusp (Fig. 10.6).

PART 2: ADULTS

Synopsis

This section provides an overview of the combined orthodontic and orthognathic treatment options in cases of severe malocclusion with underlying skeletal problems. Treatment considerations and objectives of adult orthodontic occlusion are summarised. The concepts related to postorthodontic retention – philosophy, methods and prevention of relapse – are introduced.

Key points

- The occlusion is in a constant state of biological adaptation, with age changes in the dentition, periodontal tissues and supporting structures
- Orthodontic treatment goals in adult occlusion are aimed at achieving a functionally and aesthetically acceptable occlusion within the limitations of each case. These are imposed by periodontal health, missing teeth, health of the existing teeth and general health of the individual
- More severe forms of malocclusion, such as severe mandibular retrognathia, maxillary hypoplasia, mandibular prognathism, extreme vertical dysplasia (long face syndrome), large transverse discrepancies, jaw deviations, can only be managed with

a combined orthodontic and surgical approach (orthognathic surgery). The outcome(s) are rewarding in suitable patients and require careful treatment planning
- Orthodontic treatment (including surgical orthodontic treatment) shows some relapse with time
- The severity of the relapse is governed by many factors, including the nature of the initial malocclusion, type of treatment, quality of treatment, retention protocol, residual growth of the face, type of face, presence of third molars, soft-tissue behaviour and periodontal health
- Choice of a retention appliance and specific retention protocol are governed by the type and severity of the initial malocclusion, the age of the patient and any individual predisposing factors for relapse
- Relapse is associated with and may be amplified by the natural ageing process

ADULT OCCLUSION

Adult occlusion changes continuously throughout life and adapts to intrinsic and extrinsic factors.

Physiological changes

Physiological tooth migration is the lifelong ability for teeth and their supporting tissues to adapt to functional demands and, as a result, move through the alveolar process. In humans, teeth in the posterior segments tend to migrate mesially to compensate for wear of interproximal contact surfaces. Further tooth movement may occur following changes in occlusal equilibrium with loss of a neighbouring or antagonistic tooth. In addition to mesial migration, teeth exhibit continued eruption. Studies have demonstrated continuous eruption of upper incisors by 6.0 mm per year between the ages of 19 and 25 (Iseri & Solow 1996). Growth and development of the craniofacial skeleton is a continuing, long-term process with periods of exuberance and relative quiescence, but the biological mechanisms that regulate growth changes remain intact and active throughout life.

ORTHODONTIC TREATMENT IN ADULTS

In recent years, altered lifestyles and improved dental and orthodontic awareness have led to an increased demand for orthodontic treatment by adults. The ideal treatment objectives of aesthetics, function and stability may need to be modified for adult patients, and many cases require an interdisciplinary approach. To facilitate placement of fixed or removable prostheses and a healthy periodontal status, parallelism of abutment teeth, intra-arch and interarch space distribution, adequate embrasure space and root position, and occlusal vertical dimension change need to be achieved in comprehensive treatment in conjunction with other specialities.

Aesthetics of hard and soft tissues are often the main concern for adults. The harmony of smile line, gingival level and dental alignment need to be considered as part of interdisciplinary treatment. Adults tend to be anxious about lip competency and support; many adults have a thin upper lip that may be increased in length; changes to the upper lip, with inadequate tooth, bone and soft-tissue support, create an aged appearance. The maintenance of upper lip support precludes significant retraction of maxillary incisors, and, in class II division 1, advancement of the mandibular dental arch may be the preferred treatment objective to develop incisal guidance.

Periodontal health is accomplished by improving crown : root ratio in patients who have bone loss and by correcting mucogingival and osseous defects by repositioning prominent teeth to improve gingival topography. The reduction of clinical crown length together with orthodontic extrusion will improve crown : root ratio. Location of gingival margins is determined by the axial inclination and alignment of teeth. Clinically there is improved self-maintenance of periodontal health when teeth are correctly positioned. The aim is to level crestal bone between adjacent cementoenamel junctions, as this creates a more physiological osseous architecture and the potential to correct osseous defects.

There is a delayed response to mechanical forces in adults as a result of age-related changes of the skeleton and alveolar bone. However, there is no evidence to suggest that teeth move at a slower rate. In a healthy periodontium, bone will remodel around a tooth without damage to the supporting tissues. This principle is used to create favourable alveolar bone changes in patients with periodontal defects, for example, the uprighting of molars to reduce pocket depth and improve bone morphology.

Extrusion, together with occlusal reduction of clinical crown height, is reported to reduce infrabony defects and reduce pocket depth. This procedure is advocated for the treatment of isolated periodontal osseous defects, which may be eliminated when marginal bone heights are levelled. Intrusion of teeth to improve periodontal support has been proposed, but the evidence in the literature is conflicting.

OCCLUSION AFTER TREATMENT WITH COMBINED FIXED APPLIANCE AND ORTHOGNATHIC SURGERY

Severe dysplasia of skeletal malocclusion – skeletal class II, class III or extreme open and deep bite, long face, jaw deviations – can only be corrected in a combined approach of orthodontic treatment and orthognathic surgery for surgical correction of the deformity. Where a severe skeletal class III malocclusion presents, orthodontic treatment alone is insufficient and treatment requires reduction in jaw length. A number of surgical lengthening/shortening procedures of the mandible and relocation of the maxilla are used in clinical practice. Bilateral sagittal split osteotomy (BSSO) is the most common for the mandible and Le Fort I and II (fracture of the maxilla and subsequent fixation in the required position) for the maxilla. A number of variations/combinations of occlusal relationship are governed by the type and extent of the skeletal and dental malocclusion, and the orthodontic treatment and surgical options. In general, the objectives are to provide a well-balanced harmonious face (skeletal and soft tissue), and an acceptable functioning occlusion in a class I/class II/or class III molar relationship. Ideally, the occlusion at the end of treatment should match specifications of a normal occlusion; however, depending on the severity of the discrepancy, dental compensations are accepted. Dental compensations may camouflage the extreme nature of the discrepancy in the sagittal, transverse and vertical planes.

In the sagittal plane, upper and/or lower incisors are proclined or retroclined in class II and class III orthognathic surgery cases to decrease the amount of surgical movement of the maxilla and/or mandible.

In the transverse plane, upper and/or lower posterior teeth are buccally and/or lingually tipped in posterior crossbite and buccal bite cases to decrease the amount of surgical movement of the maxilla and/or mandible.

In the vertical plane, upper and/or lower posterior teeth may be extruded or intruded; and upper and/or lower incisors may be extruded or intruded in open-bite and deep-bite cases to decrease the amount of surgical movement of the maxilla and/or mandible.

Skeletal class III These cases require shortening of the mandibular base and occasionally maxillary advancement.

Skeletal class II These cases require lengthening of the mandibular base and occasionally maxillary impaction.

ORTHODONTIC OCCLUSION IN THE LONG TERM: RELAPSE AND RETENTION

Relapse is the tendency for teeth to move from the positions in which they were placed by orthodontics, while retention is 'the holding of teeth following orthodontic treatment in the treated position for the period of time necessary for the stability of the result'.

Long-term studies of treated cases at the 10–20 year postretention period have shown that orthodontic results are potentially unstable due to:

• physiological mesial migration of teeth (age-related changes)
• periodontal and gingival health
• residual growth
• neuromuscular influences
• specific orthodontic tooth movements
• developing third molars.

A retention phase following orthodontic treatment is required to:

• allow time for periodontal and gingival reorganisation
• minimise changes in the orthodontic result from subsequent growth
• permit neuromuscular adaptation to the corrected tooth position
• maintain unstable tooth positions.

Normal developmental changes occur in the dentition in both untreated individuals and those who have undergone orthodontic treatment. The changes in the craniofacial structures, including the dental arches, are not simply due to, or the result of, orthodontic and orthopaedic treatment but are also due to ageing. There is an increase in intercanine width until eruption of the permanent canines, after which this width decreases. The intermolar

width, however, appears to be stable from 13–20 years. Mandibular arch length decreases with time and the lower incisors become increasingly irregular, particularly in females. These arch changes are observed before 30 years of age; lower incisor crowding continues beyond 50 years of age.

Periodontal and gingival tissues

The stability of tooth position is determined by the principal fibres of the periodontal ligament and the supra-alveolar gingival fibre network. These fibres contribute to a state of equilibrium between the tooth and the soft-tissue envelope. Orthodontic tooth movement causes disruption of the periodontal ligament and the gingival fibre network, and a period of time is required for reorganisation of these fibres after removal of the appliances:

• Reorganisation of the collagen fibre bundles in the periodontal ligament occurs over a 3–4 month period; at this stage tooth mobility disappears.
• The gingival fibre network is made up of both collagenous and elastic-like oxytalan fibres. Reorganisation of this network occurs more slowly than in the periodontal ligament; the collagenous fibres remodel in 4–6 months, while the oxytalan fibres may take up to 6 years to remodel.
• It is believed that the slow remodelling of the supra-alveolar fibres of the gingival complex contribute to the relapse of teeth after orthodontic treatment, especially in those teeth that were initially rotated.

The direction of relapse will tend to be towards the original position of the tooth, thus full-time retention for 3–4 months following removal of orthodontic appliances is required to allow time for reorganisation of the periodontal tissue structures. Retention should be continued part-time for at least 12 months to allow time for reorganisation of the gingival fibres.

To minimise rotational relapse, the following has been suggested:

• Early correction of the rotation to allow more time for reorganisation.
• Overcorrection of the rotation if the occlusion allows. In the premolar region overcorrection is possible, especially during early stages of the treatment. However, overcorrection at the anterior region, especially towards the achievement of the normal occlusion, when an ideal incisor relationship is obtained, is practically impossible.
• Circumferential supracrestal fibreotomy or pericision at or just before removal of appliances. This procedure involves transection of the supra-alveolar fibres, allowing reattachment in the corrected position.

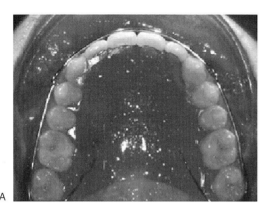
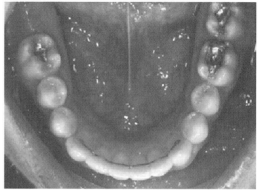

A   B

Fig. 10.7 Retention appliances. **A** Removable maxillary Begg retainer. **B** Fixed lower lingual retainer.

Neuromuscular influences

The soft tissues of the lips, cheeks and tongue at rest contribute to the equilibrium and, therefore, stability of tooth position following orthodontic treatment. The initial mandibular intercanine and intermolar arch widths are believed to be accurate indicators of the individual's muscle balance between lips, cheeks and tongue. The initial position of the lower incisor has also been shown to be the most stable position for the individual.

Permanent retention for the first 3–4 months is required to allow time for soft tissues of cheeks, lips and tongue to adapt to the new tooth positions. Wherever possible the initial intercanine width and lower incisor positions should be maintained. Permanent retention is essential if advancement of the lower incisors is an objective of treatment.

Effect of residual growth on orthodontic occlusion

Skeletal problems will tend to relapse if growth continues beyond completion of orthodontic treatment. In late adolescence, and even adulthood, continued growth in the pattern that caused a class II, class III, deep-bite or open-bite problem is a major cause of relapse and requires careful management during retention.

As a result of the residual mandibular growth, the lower incisors, contained by the upper incisors, cannot accommodate forward movement of the mandible and tend to tip lingually, causing lower incisor crowding. Clinical observation suggests finishing either with a small overjet at the end of treatment, or fixed retainers for the lower canine-to-canine area. Some clinicians rotate the mesial side of the lower canine lingually to prevent mesial movement of the canines after the retention period.

Late mandibular growth has been considered a major cause of relapse of crowding in the mandibular arch in late adulthood.

Figure 10.7 illustrates both removable and fixed retention appliances.

References

Andrews L F 1972 The six keys to normal occlusion. American Journal of Orthodontics 62:296–309

Angle E H 1906 The upper first molar as a basis of diagnosis in orthodontics. Dental Items of Interest 28:421–426

Begg P R 1954 Stone age man's dentition. American Journal of Orthodontics 40:298–312, 373–383, 462–475, 517–531

Iseri H, Solow B 1996 Continued eruption of maxillary incisors and first molars in girls from 9–25 years, studied by implant method. European Journal of Orthodontics 18:245–256

Roth R H 1981 Functional occlusion for the orthodontist. Journal of Clinical Orthodontics 15:32–51

Tweed C H 1945 A philosophy of orthodontic treatment. American Journal of Orthodontics and Oral Surgery 31:74–103

Further reading

Behrents R G 1985 An atlas of growth in the aging craniofacial skeleton. Centre for Human Growth and Development, University of Michigan, Ann Arbor, vol 18

Blake M, Bibby K 1998 Retention and stability: a review of the literature. American Journal of Orthodontics and Dentofacial Orthopedics 114:299–306

Clark J R, Evans R D 2001 Functional occlusion: a review. Journal of Orthodontics 28:76-81

Graber T M, Vanarsdall R L Jr (eds) 2000 Orthodontics: current principles and techniques, 3rd edn. Mosby, St Louis, pp 29–30

Hellman M 1920 Dental cosmos. In: Strang R H W (ed) (1950) A textbook of orthodontia, 3rd edn. Lea & Febiger, Philadelphia: p 35

Horowitz S L, Hixon E H 1969 Physiologic recovery following orthodontic treatment. American Journal of Orthodontics 55:1–4

Kasrovi P M, Meyer M, Nelson G D 2000 Occlusion: an orthodontic perspective. Journal of the California Dental Association 28:780–790

Little R M, Riedel R A, Artun J 1988 An evaluation of changes in mandibular anterior alignment from 10 to 20 years post-retention. American Journal of Orthodontics 93:423–428

Moyers R E 1988 Handbook of orthodontics, 4th edn. Chicago, Yearbook

Nangia A, Darendeliler M A 2001 Finishing occlusion in class II or class III molar relation: therapeutic class II and III. Australian Orthodontics Journal 17:89–94

Proffit W R, White R R Jr (eds) 1991 Surgical orthodontics. Mosby, St Louis, pp 248–263, 264–282

Reitan K 1960 Tissue behavior during orthodontic tooth movement. American Journal of Orthodontics 46:881–900

Richardson M E 1989 The role of the third molar in the cause of late lower arch crowding: a review. American Journal of Orthodontics and Dentofacial Orthopedics 95:79–83

Richardson M E 1999 Prophylactic extraction of lower third molars: setting the record straight. American Journal of Orthodontics and Dentofacial Orthopedics 115(1):17A–18A

Richardson M E 1999 A review of changes in lower arch alignment from seven to fifty years. Seminars in Orthodontics 5:151–159

Richardson M E, Gormley J S 1998 Lower arch crowding in the third decade. European Journal of Orthodontics 20:597–607

Roth R H 1987 The straight wire appliance 17 years later. Journal of Clinical Orthodontics 21: 632–642

Staley R N 2001 In: Bishara S E (ed) Text book of orthodontics. Saunders, Philadelphia, pp 98–104

Strang R H W 1950 A Textbook of orthodontia, 2nd edn. Lea & Febiger, Philadelphia, pp 24–51, 78–106

Thilander B 2000 Orthodontic relapse versus natural development. American Journal of Orthodontics and Dentofacial Orthopedics 117:562–563

Vaden J L, Dale J G, Klontz H A 2000 The Tweed–Merrifield appliance: philosophy, diagnosis and treatment. In: Graber T M, Vanarsdall R L Jr (eds) Orthodontics: current principles and techniques, 3rd edn. Mosby, St Louis, pp 647–707

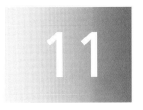

11

Occlusion and fixed prosthodontics

T. Walton

Synopsis

This chapter presents the rationale for establishing tooth contact patterns during fixed prosthodontic procedures, i.e. for establishing a therapeutic occlusal form.

In the absence of scientific data, various 'philosophies of occlusion' have evolved in an effort to describe the relationships that should be developed between the teeth during restorative procedures or adjustment of the natural dentition. With little evidence, these philosophies or concepts often involve complicated and expensive instrumentation and some are promoted with almost religious zeal rather than scientific rigor.

Form that supports function is the basis of the rationale for occlusal form outlined in this chapter. The biological, physiological and mechanical results of an up-to-15-year longitudinal assessment of the outcome of single crowns and fixed partial dentures provides evidence for its effectiveness.

There is a need for further long-term studies evaluating the outcome of fixed prosthodontics. It is accepted that prospective, randomised clinical trials with adequate controls and well-defined criteria are very difficult to carry out. In addition, clinical studies of less than 5 years have little relevance (Cruegers et al 1994) and can lead to incorrect conclusions (Walton 2002). It is therefore imperative that clinicians document and publish information from their clinical practice. The resultant collective data would facilitate a more evidence-based approach to procedures used in fixed prosthodontics.

Key points

The following are the key points for establishing occlusal form in fixed prosthodontics.
- Intra-arch stability effected by firm interproximal contacts
- Interarch stability effected by at least one contact on each opposing tooth in ICP
- Bilateral synchronised contacts in ICP
- Absence of posterior contacts during protrusive movements
- A flat occlusal plane
- Maintenance of physiological tooth mobility where possible
- Slight clearance (10 μm foil thickness) between the incisors in maximum intercuspation (MI)
- Minimal cusp height and fossa depth
- Lateral gliding contacts restricted to the canines or effected as far forward in the arch as possible

INTRODUCTION

Occlusion is the dynamic interplay of various components including the teeth, their supporting tissues, the jaw muscles, the temporomandibular joints and the central pattern generator and other associated cortical interactions. As in any physiological system, a 'normal' state includes a degree of adaptability with a range of form and the absence of pathology. The magnitude of any changes and the duration over which they occur will influence whether adaptation or pathology ensues. Slow changes will facilitate adaptation even when the changes eventually lead to a significant deviation from ideal form. Fixed prosthodontics, however, involves relatively instantaneous changes in form, thus challenging the adaptive capacity of the occlusal system. A therapeutic occlusal form that requires minimal adaptation will be less likely to initiate pathology, and the health of the occlusal components will be determined to a great extent by the subsequent stability of the teeth.

TOOTH CONTACTS

There has been debate regarding the number and position of contacts required to maintain individual tooth stability. Contacts on natural teeth occur on flat surfaces, marginal ridges, cusp tips, cusp inclines and in fossa. They may be point or plane contacts. Philosophies of occlusion that prescribe specific and multiple point per tooth contact patterns assume a required precision that does not occur naturally. It has not been demonstrated that such precision results in any greater long-term stability of tooth position than that which occurs in the natural unrestored dentition.

Contacts between teeth result in vertical and lateral forces and significant tipping and rotations may occur if tooth position is unstable. Maintaining interproximal contacts facilitates intra-arch stability while inter-arch tooth stability is facilitated by bilateral contacts between opposing teeth in the intercuspal position (ICP). However, the relatively short time that opposing teeth contact indicates that other forces arising from the tongue and facial musculature, the periodontal ligament and alveolar bone transceptal fibres may also influence long-term tooth stability.

FORM THAT SUPPORTS FUNCTION

The functions performed by components of the occlusion include suckling, swallowing, speech, mastication and para-function. They also contribute to self-image (aesthetics) and emotional expression.

Suckling

Suckling is an innate reflex that does not involve the teeth. However, in its mature form sucking might be considered a parafunction if habits such as finger or tongue sucking become prolonged. The forces involved during such para-function and other habits, such as tongue thrusting, can affect the position and stability of the teeth, especially those with reduced periodontal support, and may be linked to specific skeletal jaw morphology. Therefore, although these forces have little bearing on considerations of tooth form in fixed prosthodontics, it is important to recognise their existence when assessing and effecting long-term follow-up. For example the overcontoured palatal form of a crowned maxillary central incisor in conjunction with a tongue-thrust habit may result in mobility or migration of the tooth even in the absence of any opposing tooth contact.

Swallowing

Swallowing is also an innate reflex response, that does not necessarily involve the teeth. An important aspect of swallowing involves bracing of the jaw to support the suprahyoid muscles. This is achieved during the infantile swallow pattern by bracing the tongue against the palate. Although the tongue is sometimes used for jaw bracing by children and adults, for example when drinking, the more common means of jaw bracing during swallowing involves contact between the teeth in ICP. The forces involved are relatively light. Thus contact between only a few teeth would be unlikely to involve excessive loading leading to symptoms within the teeth or periodontal tissues. Tooth contacts during swallowing will also vary with head posture. The occlusal form of the teeth and their interarch contacts would seem to have little bearing on swallowing. However, bilateral synchronised tooth contacts at ICP may facilitate optimum physiological neuromuscular activity during swallowing.

Phonetics

The arrangement of the anterior teeth will affect phonetics as well as aesthetics. The proximity of the upper and lower anterior teeth during protrusive movements, for example, will determine the 'c', 's' and 't' sounds. The relationship of the upper anterior teeth and the lip will affect 'f' and 'v' sounds. As well as facilitating inter-personal communication, there is a social expectation that phonetic patterns will be effected in a specific way. Thus, the absence of anterior teeth, or any impediment such as posterior contacts that prevent anterior tooth approximation when protruding the jaw for speech, can affect self-image as well as speech.

Excessive lateral deviation or torquing around posterior teeth to develop socially acceptable speech patterns will require adaptation of the jaw neuromuscular system. Exceeding the physiological 'adaptability' of one or more of these components may result in pain or dysfunction. The length of the incisors, the degree of overbite and overjet, the angle of condylar inclination and the curve of the occlusal plane will influence anterior tooth approximation during protrusion. These factors, except condylar inclination, may be modified by restorative procedures. Tooth form and tooth arrangement should therefore ensure an absence of posterior contacts during protrusive jaw movements and this will be facilitated by developing a flat occlusal plane. Thus restorative procedures, which influence phonetics, may also affect the patient's psycho-logical and physiological well-being.

Mastication

Mastication usually involves an approximation but not necessarily contact between posterior teeth. It is possible to prepare a food bolus for swallowing without tooth contact. The efficiency of comminution of the food bolus will be influenced by the contour of the occlusal surfaces. Steep cuspal inclines may or may not promote chewing efficiency but will increase lateral loading on the teeth. The need for chewing efficiency (and posterior teeth) has decreased significantly with modern food-handling techniques. Thus the actual occlusal form provided during restorative procedures would seem to have minimal effect on mastication. The effect of lateral loading on teeth may be more significant, especially if the restored teeth have reduced periodontal and bony support. In these circumstances low cusp height and shallow fossa depth appear to be beneficial to reduce lateral loads.

Parafunction

Tooth clenching and grinding (bruxing) are common forms of parafunction involving tooth contacts. However, it may be difficult to distinguish between what is normal physiological activity and what is parafunctional activity. Clenching during power activities such as weight lifting is more likely a normal physiological action than parafunction. Clenching and bruxing during tooth eruption or during stress may also be part of normal physiological activity. It is generally agreed that forces generated during these activities are greater than during other forms of tooth contact. It is likely that these forms of parafunction are universal. Their amplitude and frequency, however, vary significantly between individuals and result in various forms of adaptability and morphological changes including muscular hyperthrophy, tooth movement, tooth intrusion and wear, periodontal ligament thickening, increased periodontal bone density and temporomandibular joint (TMJ) remodelling. They may possibly also result in pathological changes, including neuromuscular and TMJ dysfunction, tooth and periodontal ligament sensitivity and pulpal inflammation.

It should be assumed that all patients at some time engage in tooth clenching and grinding, either physiological or parafunctional, and that dental restorations will be subjected to the relatively high magnitude of forces involved. It therefore seems prudent to apply an occlusal scheme that promotes the integrity of the occlusal components assuming the presence of such forces.

TOOTH WEAR

Tooth wear by itself cannot be considered a pathological consequence of parafunctional activity. Only when the rate of wear exceeds the response of the pulp and results in pain can it be considered pathological. However, tooth wear and increased tooth mobility may become psychologically debilitating and socially unacceptable. There are cultural differences between what is considered acceptable tooth wear, as there are cultural differences in what is considered acceptable tooth colour. Just as commercial marketing has promoted the concept that all teeth should be 'white', there is a perception that teeth should maintain their adolescent form throughout life.

MAINTAINING TOOTH INTEGRITY

The periodontal ligament is structured to convert compressive forces to tensile strain between the tooth and supporting bone and does this most efficiently when the forces are applied along the long axes of the teeth. Bone resorbs under compression, but its structural integrity is stimulated under moderate tensile forces. The inherent resilience imparted by the periodontal ligament acts as a shock absorber during the application of force, thus lowering the impact loads that have to be sustained by bone, teeth and restorative materials. In addition, movement of the teeth away from an applied force can allow other teeth to accept the load. Initial contact in or around ICP is often limited to one or two teeth, but as the biting force increases, more teeth accept the load (Riise & Ericsson 1983). Thus physiological tooth mobility is a 'protective' mechanism and helps to ensure tooth and bone integrity. It will also help preserve the mechanical integrity of restorations. Splinting of teeth may be necessary but maintaining individual tooth mobility where possible rather than joining teeth together for restorative purposes would seem to be a worthwhile goal. The use of non-rigid connection in fixed partial dentures may assist in achieving this goal and help maintain the mechanical integrity of any prosthesis (Walton 2003).

Excessive lateral loading can result in structural failure of teeth (fracture) or breakdown of supporting structures. Teeth that are structurally weakened through dental caries and resultant restorative procedures, or have lost support through periodontal disease, are particularly affected by increased lateral loading. Forces applied to the teeth during clenching and grinding will be higher than those applied during any other function. Thus the loading on tooth form and contacts developed during restorative treatment will be greatest during parafunction. Lateral loading should be minimised to ensure biological health and mechanical integrity.

The maxillary anterior teeth are most likely to be subjected to increased lateral loading during clenching and chewing because of their inclination (Wiskott & Belser 1995). This will be further exacerbated following posterior tooth wear (and possibly restoration) and any associated loss in occlusal vertical dimension (OVD). Excessive contact between the anterior teeth results in fremitus when closing into the intercuspal position. Anterior flaring may also occur if excessive anterior tooth contact prevails over a long period, especially if there is associated loss in periodontal support. Splinting of teeth may reduce fremitus, but because of its limiting effect on inherent tooth mobility it may also increase tooth fracture. Tooth fracture has been shown to be the most common form of failure associated with fixed partial dentures (Walton 2003). Given that it is not possible to measure the intensity of contacts clinically, it would seem prudent to establish and maintain slight clearance (10 μm foil thickness) between the anterior teeth in ICP.

All teeth are potentially subjected to increased lateral loading during eccentric bruxism. It is assumed that the shallower the cuspal inclines and fossae, the less lateral loading will be developed during gliding tooth contacts.

LATERAL TOOTH GUIDANCE DURING FUNCTION

Canine teeth are well adapted to accept lateral loading (Ch. 1). They have a favourable crown : root ratio; are broad buccolingually; are encased in dense and well-buttressed bone; and the cuspal inclination is relatively shallow. In other animals the canine is most laterally loaded during tearing of food. This evolutionary adaptation is redundant in humans for food gathering, but has established the canine as capable of withstanding lateral forces involved in parafunction. This fact can be utilised in restorative procedures. Unless the canine is structurally weakened, or canine contact is not possible during eccentric movements (Angle class II division 1 anterior tooth arrangement), it appears to be reasonable to concentrate lateral gliding contacts on the canines during restorative procedures. When this is not possible it is clinically prudent to distribute lateral forces over several teeth, but furthest away from the point of application of maximum biting force, that is, as far forward in the arch as possible. When canine guidance is not possible then eccentric gliding contacts may be distributed simultaneously over several teeth i.e. 'group function' involving incisors and premolars to distribute lateral forces on less biomechanically robust teeth.

Posterior teeth may act as pivoting fulcrum points during gliding movements. This may result in distraction and negative pressure within the ipsilateral TMJ in association with tensile stress on capsular attachments, as suggested by Hylander (1979). Repeated stress may lead to strain involving stretching or tearing of the attachments

and result in 'looseness' in the joint. This may affect condylar movements. Developing a flat occlusal plane will help to avoid posterior eccentric contacts.

SUPPORTING EVIDENCE FROM CLINICAL OUTCOME STUDIES

As a result of these considerations, the factors above are proposed recommendations for establishing tooth form and contacts during restorative procedures. There are no prospective studies confirming that a particular design promotes physiological and mechanical stability in fixed prosthodontic treatment. There are few longitudinal outcome studies that detail the occlusal contact pattern used as part of the study protocol. However, a retrospective 10-year review of single crowns and fixed partial dentures incorporating the above recommendations into the treatment protocol resulted in only 2% of 344 patients developing temporomandibular dysfunction (TMD) subsequent to treatment (Walton 1997). Of these patients, 78% had experienced TMD before treatment and the development of post-treatment symptoms may have been part of the cyclical nature of TMD. In addition only 0.5% of 688 metal–ceramic single unit crowns up to 10 years (Walton 1999) and 0.1% of 1208 abutments in 515 metal–ceramic fixed partial dentures up to 15 years (Walton 2002, 2003) mechanically failed (lost retention, fracture of the materials). These data suggest that the guidelines for occlusal form as described above contributed to physiological and mechanical stability.

HARM VERSUS BENEFIT

Dental treatment involves a degree of iatrogenic injury. The benefits of dental restoration must therefore be weighed against the injury caused. In the absence of signs or symptoms of dysfunction associated with the occlusion, or compromised tooth structure integrity, or poor aesthetics (teeth or supporting structures), it is difficult to justify any restorative procedures (or occlusal adjustment). Cultural demands to restore tooth wear, discoloration or other perceived tooth imperfections and even tooth replacement may result in overtreatment, where the benefits are outweighed by the iatrogenic consequences or financial costs of the procedures and necessary long-term maintenance. The concept of 'the shortened dental arch' as a viable treatment option had its genesis in the reality that tooth replacement in the posterior segments often results in iatrogenic injury to remaining hard and soft tissues without significant improvement in function.

THE 'CENTRIC' TREATMENT POSITION

There has been much confusion and debate regarding the correct maxillomandibular relationship (MMR) to be utilised during restorative procedures. Initial consideration of MMR was applied to the construction of complete dentures where there were no naturally occurring interdental relationships. Jaw closure around the TMJs at a specific vertical dimension was the reference point, and instrumentation was developed to simulate this arc of closure. The actual position of the condyle in the glenoid fossa became a controversial topic (Ch. 1).

Recording retruded jaw position (RP) or centric relation (CR) has also been a contentious issue. Jaw guidance by the dentist to ensure correct condyle–fossa relationships has been strongly advocated by some clinicians. However, it is difficult to assess what guidance force should be applied to the resilient TMJs to prevent a strained joint position. In addition, different operators will inevitably apply different guiding force. It is difficult to accept that a physiological MMR would be obtained. Furthermore, to assess when the condyles are in a 'desired' position in the fossae is not clinically possible. Other clinicians advocate a non-guided closure, provided that deflective tooth contacts are either absent or eliminated. However, in this case it is difficult to assess if habitual neuromuscular patterns mask the optimum physiological closure path and possibly perpetuate recording of a strained TMJ relationship. Interarch recording materials that eliminate tooth contacts can be utilised to relate casts in RP at a given OVD. Further opening or closure of articulated casts along this arc will only represent the clinical situation if the hinge axis has been determined and the orientation of the casts in relation to the hinge axis is identical to that which occurs clinically.

Intercuspal contact position will be determined in part by biting force and head posture. Following initial contact the tooth surfaces may cause a deviation in the arc of closure and individual tooth movement may result in more teeth contacting as bite force increases. Indeed, it is well established (Ch. 1) that only about 10% of the population have an ICP that is coincident with RCP clinically.

Maximum interdigitation of teeth on casts is repeatable for a given set of casts, but will be determined by the position of the teeth recorded in the impressions. In most instances it will very closely simulate the clinical ICP resulting with moderate biting force. It is a convenient and acceptable reference for indirect restorative procedures, provided that individual teeth have minimal mobility and there are sufficient tooth contacts to stabilise the casts. Deflective tooth contacts may result in this reference position being anterior or lateral to the MMR in RP (CR).

The recorded maximum interdigitation of teeth on casts should be used for single tooth restorations, fixed partial dentures involving one or unilateral posterior teeth, or fixed partial dentures involving anterior tooth restoration or replacement. This assumes an absence of either signs or symptoms of dysfunction or a significant deviation (>2.0 mm) from the RCP position,

Tooth contact relationships may be altered by occlusal adjustment or by changes to the contour of provisional restorations and may result in an area of possible tooth contacts rather than point contacts. The resultant contact area may include the ICP position at the same vertical dimension. There is no scientific evidence to specify that such an adjustment is necessary before carrying out restorative procedures. It may be indicated to enhance individual tooth integrity where contacts occur on inclines of teeth that have become structurally weakened by previous restorative procedures. Occlusal adjustment (Ch. 15) may then result in a reduction in the lateral component of the applied force.

ROLE OF INSTRUMENTATION

Instruments used in fixed prosthodontics should allow development of a physiological occlusion and should not require a specific tooth contact pattern. Irrespective of the degree of sophistication of the instrumentation, harmony of the various occlusal components must be established. It is prudent to simplify the role and type of any instrumentation employed, given the possibilities for inaccuracies developing in the many procedures involved (Ch. 6).

Changes to the occlusal form during restorative procedures may preclude the use of ICP as a treatment position. Prior elimination of deflective tooth contacts by occlusal adjustment or with the use of provisional restorations would be likely to unmask any habitual neuromuscular patterns. Subsequently, a patient-directed recording would probably result in a physiological RCP and avoid the variables associated with active jaw guidance by the clinician. Recording the MMR at the anticipated restored OVD then eliminates the need to record the hinge axis accurately. It has been claimed, however, that when an arbitrary hinge axis is used, rotational changes of the articulated casts of up to 2 mm (measured at the teeth) will not induce errors above clinically tolerable levels (Morneburg & Pröschel 2002). Providing the recording medium itself does not cause jaw deflection, the subsequently restored tooth contact pattern (ICP) will approach CO.

The need to record and reproduce lateral jaw movements accurately can be eliminated by restricting lateral gliding contact patterns between as few teeth as possible, minimising cusp height and fossa depth, and developing a flat occlusal plane. Average value settings on an articulator may be appropriate to ensure adequate clearance of posterior teeth during lateral movements. A facebow oriented along an arbitrary hinge axis is a convenient method for locating casts relative to the inter-condylar axis through the condyle spheres of an articulator. Further, this can closely simulate the actual position of the jaws in the frontal, sagittal and vertical planes relative to the TMJs. A flat occlusal plane indicator may be just as effective for some clinical procedures (Shodadai et al 2001). It has been mathematically derived that when average value articulator settings are used there is a relatively low risk of inducing occlusal errors at premolar and molar regions during lateral movements (Pröschel & Morneburg 2000). Thus, even if group function involving posterior teeth is indicated (e.g. Angle class II division 1 tooth relationships), only minor intraoral adjustment would be necessary to ensure appropriate tooth contacts.

There are no published data validating improved outcomes in fixed prosthodontics when complex jaw movement recording devices and fully adjustable articulators are used. On the other hand, use of instrumentation as described in this chapter for fixed prosthodontic treatment has been found to be appropriate to ensure optimum outcome of prostheses up to 15 years (Walton 2002). There has also been minimal physiological disharmony of the occlusal components in monitoring patient treatments for up to 10 years (Walton 1999).

OCCLUSAL PLANE ORIENTATION

Emphasis in the past was given to the orientation of the occlusal plane. Initial consideration related to the stability of complete dentures by minimising the posterior space between the appliances in eccentric movements. The compensating curves (curve of Spee and curve of Wilson) facilitated a balanced occlusion for a given anterior overjet and overbite. Other concepts like the Monson curves have been used to orient the occlusal plane in fixed prostheses to develop multiple contacts in eccentric movements such as group function. There is no evidence that there is any relationship between occlusal plane orientation and either function or outcome of fixed prostheses.

In the natural dentition the most significant feature of the occlusal plane relates to aesthetics rather than function. The anteroposterior cant, measured by reference to the incisal edges and buccal cusp tips of the maxillary teeth, mostly follows the curve of the lower lip when in the smile pose and this has an association with a pleasing appearance. Thus a 'steep' cant will often be associated

with an Angle class II skeletal pattern and an obtuse gonial angle. A flat curve is often associated with a more acute gonial angle. Where it is possible to change the orientation of the occlusal plane in fixed prosthodontics, it should be related to aesthetic rather than any perceived functional considerations.

LONG TERM MAINTENANCE

The recommendations outlined in this chapter are designed to result in relative stability of the dentition to minimise adaptation and/or the development of pathology. It is accepted that changes will inevitably occur with time, and minor changes in tooth position, even in intact arches, have been demonstrated. Differential wear between anterior and posterior teeth will occur due to the varying forces applied. Many dentitions will have several materials (natural and artificial) forming occlusal contacts, and different toughness, abrasion- and erosion-resistant properties will result in differential wear of these materials. Long-term monitoring of the teeth and supporting structures should include adjustments to maintain the described contact patterns for maximising biological, physiological and mechanical stability.

 References

Creugers N H, Kayser A F, van't Hof M A 1994 A meta-analysis of durability data on conventional fixed bridges. Community Dentistry and Oral Epidemiology 22:448–452

Hylander W L 1979 An experimental analysis of temporomandibular joint reaction force in macaques. American Journal of Physical Anthropology 51:433–456

Morneburg T R , Pröschel P A 2002 Predicted incidence of occlusal errors in centric closing around arbitrary axes. International Journal of Prosthodontics 15:358–364.

Pröschel P A, Maul T, Morneburg T R 2000 Predicted incidence of excursive occlusal errors in common modes of articulator adjustment. International Journal of Prosthodontics 13:303–310

Riise C, Ericsson S G 1983 A clinical study of the distribution of occlusal tooth contacts in the intercuspal position in light and hard pressure in adults. Journal of Oral Rehabilitation 10:473–480

Shodadai S P, Türp J C, Gerds T, Strub J R 2001 Is there a benefit of using an arbitrary facebow for the fabrication of a stabilization appliance? International Journal of Prosthodontics 14:517–522

Walton T R 1997 A ten-year longitudinal study of fixed prosthodontics: 1. Protocol and patient profile. International Journal of Prosthodontics 10:325–331

Walton T R 1999 A 10-year longitudinal study of fixed prosthodontics: clinical characteristics and outcome of single-unit metal–ceramic crowns. International Journal of Prosthodontics 12:519–526

Walton T R 2002 An up to 15-year study of 515 metal–ceramic fixed partial dentures: Part 1. Outcome. International Journal of Prosthodontics 15:439–445

Walton T R 2003 An up to 15-year study of 515 metal–ceramic fixed partial dentures: Part 2. Modes of failure and influence of various clinical characteristics. International Journal of Prosthodontics (in press)

Wiskott H W, Belser U C 1995 A rationale for a simplified occlusal design in restorative dentistry: historical review and clinical guidelines. Journal of Prosthetic Dentistry 73:169–183

Further reading

Beyron H L 1969 Optimal occlusion. Dental Clinics of North America 13:537–554

Helsing G, Helsing E, Eliasson S 1995 The hinge axis concept: a radiographic study of its relevance. Journal of Prosthetic Dentistry 73:60–64

Picton D C 1962 Tilting movements of teeth during biting. Archives of Oral Biology 7:151–159

Sarver D M 2001 The importance of incisor positioning in the esthetic smile: the smile arc. American Journal of Orthodontics and Dentofacial Orthopedics 120:98–111

Tradowsky M, Kubicek W F 1981 Method for determining the physiologic equilibrium point of the mandible. Journal of Prosthetic Dentistry 45:558–563

Wood G N 1998 Centric relation and the treatment position in rehabilitating occlusions: a physiologic approach. Part 2: The treatment position. Journal of Prosthetic Dentistry 60:15–18

12 Occlusion and removable prosthodontics

R. Jagger

Synopsis

Occlusal considerations for removable prostheses are essentially the same as for fixed restorations.

The approach to establishing occlusion for removable partial dentures is usually conformative. Partial dentures should not transmit excessive forces to supporting tissues nor interfere with any contacts in intercuspal position or in functional movements. Occasionally a reconstructive approach using onlays is used.

Occlusion for complete dentures has three significant differences:

- The absence of natural teeth in edentulous patients may present significant difficulties in determining an acceptable occlusal vertical dimension.
- Complete denture occlusion is always a reorganised occlusion.
- Absence of teeth produces problems of denture stability (resistance to displacement by lateral forces), particularly of the mandibular complete denture. The stability of complete dentures is optimised by a balanced occlusion/articulation.

This chapter provides an overview of occlusion for partial and complete removable prostheses, including discussion of both clinical and laboratory procedures.

Key points

- Partial dentures
  - Occlusion: conformative/reorganised approaches
  - Treatment planning for partial dentures

- Occlusal analysis
- Clinical stages
- Onlay dentures
- Complete dentures
  - Occlusion for complete dentures
  - Occlusal vertical dimension
  - Artificial teeth
  - Balanced occlusion
  - Lingualised occlusion
  - Occlusion and patient satisfaction
  - Clinical stages

Good occlusal practice for removable dentures is very similar to that described for fixed prostheses.

Partial dentures should not transmit excessive forces to supporting tissues nor interfere in intercuspal position or in functional movements. The occlusal form is usually conformative with the natural teeth. Occasionally a reconstructive approach using onlays is used. Occlusion for complete dentures, however, has three significant differences:

- The absence of natural teeth in edentulous patients may present significant difficulties in determining an acceptable occlusal vertical dimension (OVD).
- Complete denture occlusion is always a 'reorganised' occlusion.
- Absence of teeth produces problems of denture stability (resistance to displacement by lateral forces), particularly of the mandibular complete denture. The stability of complete dentures is optimised by a balanced occlusion.

PARTIAL DENTURES

Occlusion: conformative / reorganised

The usual goal of partial denture treatment (in respect of the occlusion) is to position the artificial teeth so that there is even contact and maximum intercuspation (MI) in the intercuspal position (ICP). For more extensive partial dentures, such as bilateral distal extension saddle dentures, the aim might also be to achieve a balanced occlusion.

Occasionally, instead of this conformative approach a reorganised approach is used when onlays or an onlay appliance covers some or all of the occluding surfaces of the dental arch.

Treatment planning for partial dentures

When replacing missing teeth, it is of evident importance that treatment is based on a comprehensive treatment plan. The treatment plan must be derived from a careful history, examination and the use of appropriate special investigations. For the partially dentate patient, special investigations include radiographs, tooth vitality tests and usually articulated, surveyed study casts. The treatment plan for the partially dentate patient must include a detailed design of any prosthesis.

Occlusal analysis

During the treatment-planning phase it is important to analyse the occlusion to detect any tooth alignment problems, such as overeruption, that might prevent the construction of a prosthesis with a satisfactory occlusion. A decision must be made as to whether any preprosthetic occlusal adjustments or alterations are necessary; for example, the removal of any tooth cusp interferences along the arc of closure into ICP. Occlusal analysis is done both in the mouth and by the use of articulated study casts.

A detailed account of clinical occlusal analysis has been given in Chapter 5.

Study casts may be articulated without an occlusal record if intercuspal position is coincident with centric relation (CR) and if there are sufficient teeth to provide stable intercuspation of study casts. If there are insufficient teeth, wax occlusal rims are usually used to determine centric jaw relation (CR).

Clinical stages

Recording centric jaw relation

The working casts also may be articulated without an occlusal record if centric occlusion (CO) is coincident with CR and if there are sufficient teeth to provide stable ICP of the casts, If there are insufficient teeth, wax occlusal rims are used. The wax may be placed on shellac or acrylic base plates, or more commonly on the metal framework. If the wax rims are to be placed on the framework it is important to ensure beforehand that the framework fits accurately and does not interfere with the occlusion in retruded contact position (RCP, ICP) or in lateral excursions.

Insertion – occlusal correction

Minor interferences are often present, as in complete dentures, due to previous clinical or laboratory errors. The dentures must be adjusted so that the natural teeth meet in precisely the same way both with and without the dentures in place.

Often chairside adjustment by selective grinding is sufficient. Marks produced by articulating paper must be interpreted with caution, by visual confirmation and by asking the patient for his or her perception of how the teeth contact. The patient should be asked whether the teeth contact evenly or meet on one side first. If aware of a premature contact, can the patient feel which tooth or teeth meet first. Again, this information must be used with caution.

When maxillary and mandibular dentures are being inserted, each denture must be checked and corrected separately. A final correction is done with both dentures in place.

Very occasionally the occlusal errors are so large that chairside correction is not possible. In these cases, the artificial teeth causing the interferences should be ground off. Wax can be placed on the base in those regions and CR can be rerecorded. If the denture has been returned to the clinic with the casts, a new occlusal record can be taken, the casts remounted and the occlusion corrected in the laboratory. Otherwise an overall impression should be taken with the denture(s) in place. The impressions should be cast and the dentures rearticulated, reset and retried.

Onlay/overlay dentures

Whereas complete dentures always have a reorganised occlusion, partial dentures usually have a 'conformative' occlusion.

A reorganised approach for partial dentures may be considered:

- to correct an overclosed occlusion
- to improve the occlusion, for example when there is a gross discrepancy between RCP and the intercuspal position.

This approach is achieved by the use of onlays.

When a component of the partial denture extends to cover the greater proportion of the occlusal or incisal surface of a tooth it is called an onlay or overlay. Onlays may be used to cover one, many or all of the teeth in the dental arch. They may be made of acrylic resin or cast-metal denture base materials. An alternative method is to add acrylic resin onto retention tags in metal that has been cast to the fitting surface of the teeth. This has the advantage that the occlusal surface may be easily adjusted.

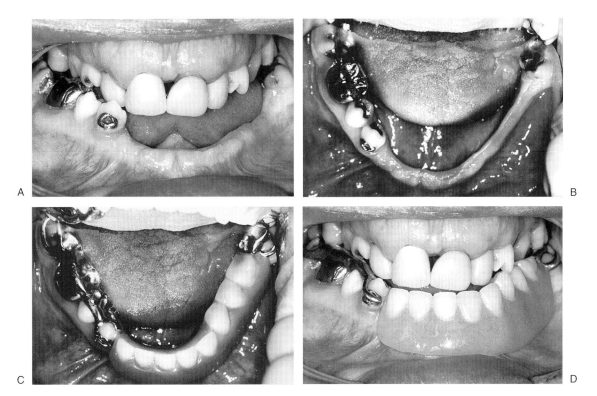

Fig. 12.1   A–D A mandibular partial onlay denture. The appliance replaces one of similar design that had been worn for approximately 20 years.

Diagnostic or temporary onlays are usually constructed in acrylic resin.

The use of an onlay appliance to correct an overclosed occlusion is shown in Figure 12.1.

Extensive coverage of teeth by occlusal onlays can predispose to dental caries. If clinical conditions allow, fixed restorations are the preferred treatment.

COMPLETE DENTURES

Occlusion

In a detailed overview of the literature of occlusal considerations in complete dentures, Palla (1997) noted that patients' satisfaction with complete dentures is a complex phenomenon and that the occlusion plays only a minor part. Further, there is little evidence to support commonly held views on the advantages or disadvantages of tooth form, tooth arrangement or occlusal schemes.

Patient satisfaction with dentures does not correlate closely with technical quality. For example, patients with greatly decreased vertical dimension and severely worn occlusal surfaces may have no complaint about their dentures. Indeed they may be unable to adapt to new

'better' dentures. Nevertheless, it is important to understand the principles of occlusion related to removable prostheses in order to try to provide optimum treatment best suited to each individual. The clinician should have a clear picture of the occlusion that he or she is trying to achieve for each patient.

Recommended occlusion for complete dentures

- Recommended practice is to develop *maximum intercuspation of complete dentures to coincide with CR at an acceptable OVD*. Failure to achieve that can lead to intolerance, usually because of instability of the dentures or because of pain of the alveolar mucosa as a result of uneven load distribution and high stress concentrations.
- It is also recommended that a *balanced occlusion* (i.e. harmonious contacts between maxillary and mandibular teeth in all excursive movements) is provided in order to help give occlusal stability.

Occlusal vertical dimension

There is much evidence to show that it is possible to increase OVD without adverse consequences, in both the natural dentition and in complete dentures (Palla 1997).

There are limits to an individual's ability to adapt to opening or closing an OVD. The OVD has a great influence on facial appearance. Complete dentures with insufficient freeway space cause difficulties with speech and may result in pain beneath the denture.

It can be very difficult to determine an acceptable correct OVD once it is lost and many methods have been developed to help establish OVD (Table 12.1). These are described in detail in standard prosthetic dentistry texts. Perhaps the most commonly used method has been to determine postural jaw position (PJP, 'resting vertical dimension'). OVD is then established 2–4 mm less than PJP. PJP is not constant, however, and methods used to

measure it generally have poor reproducibility. It varies with, among other things, head posture, the instructions given to the patient to achieve 'rest' and with time. It is also known that altering an OVD will lead to the establishment of a new PJP.

The clinician must register an OVD and pass that information to the technician. Experienced clinicians usually rely on a combination of methods at the registration stage; for example, measuring PJP, observing patient appearance at selected OVD and measuring the OVD of previously satisfactory dentures. Clinicians must then try to verify the dimension at try-in stage, again by the use of a similar combination of methods.

It is usually possible to provide a patient with new dentures with a greater OVD than that of the previous old dentures. It is wise to test any increase by the progressive addition of autopolymerising acrylic to the occlusal surfaces of the artificial teeth of the old dentures.

Artificial teeth

Artificial teeth are made from either acrylic resin or porcelain. The quality of acrylic teeth has improved greatly in recent years and porcelain teeth are no longer commonly used.

Two types of posterior cusp form are produced by manufacturers of artificial teeth (Fig. 12.2):

- Anatomical teeth – may have different cuspal angulations, e.g. 20°, 30° or 40° cuspal angle; 20° cuspal angle teeth are commonly used for complete dentures.

Table 12.1 Some methods used to determine occlusal vertical dimension

- Postural position (PJP, resting vertical dimension); OVD is approximately 2–4 mm less
- Measure OVD of satisfactory previous dentures
- Aesthetics
- Ridge parallelism: Paralleling the crests of maxillary and mandibular edentulous ridges plus a 5° posterior opening gives an indication of correct vertical dimension.
- Pre-extraction records
- Lateral skull radiographs
- Facial measurement
- Phonetics
- Patient reported position of comfort
- Intraoral central bearing pin

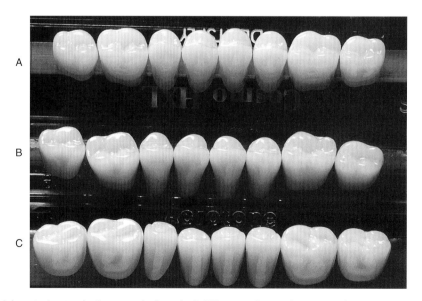

Fig. 12.2 Artificial posterior teeth. **A** anatomical teeth; **B** 10° cusps; **C** zero degree teeth.

- Zero-degree teeth (flat-cusped, cuspless) – are said to be indicated for cases with flat alveolar ridges or where there is great difficulty recording CR.

Research has not provided evidence to support commonly held views on advantages and disadvantages of artificial tooth form. For example, while it is possible that selection of artificial posterior teeth, such as cusped rather than cuspless, may have a marginal effect on chewing efficiency, other factors, in particular retention and stability of the dentures, have far more effect.

Balanced occlusion

Balanced occlusion refers to occlusion with simultaneous contacts of the occlusal surface of all or some of the teeth on both sides of the arch in all mandibular positions. A balanced occlusion is developed by the dental technician on the articulator.

The five determinants or variables affecting occlusal contacts are known as Hanau's quint:

1. *Orientation of occlusal plane.* Average-value articulators have preset distances between the condylar components and the incisal tips. The orientation of the occlusal plane is determined by the clinician when trimming the upper occlusal rim.
2. *Condylar guidance.* Condylar angles of average value articulators are also preset, usually at 30°.
3. *Incisal guidance.* Incisal guidance is commonly set arbitrarily at 10 or 15°.
4. *Cuspal angle.* The cuspal angles of the artificial teeth are produced by the manufacturer.
5. *Compensating curve.* The dental technician sets the artificial teeth with a compensating curve that allows for a balanced occlusion.

The extent to which the balanced occlusion/articulation developed on an articulator will be present in the mouth will depend on the accuracy of the centric jaw registration used to articulate the casts. It will also depend on the degree to which the settings of the articulator replicate the corresponding parameters of the patient's jaws. Use of a semiadjustable articulator and a facebow record, and lateral and protrusive records to set condylar angles, will more accurately replicate the mouth than an average value articulator. In most cases when inserting dentures it will be necessary to adjust the occlusion, for example using articulating foil in the mouth and specific occlusal adjustment at the chairside, in order to produce a balanced occlusion.

Lingualised occlusion

In conventional artificial tooth arrangement the lower artificial buccal cusps occlude with the fossae of the opposing upper teeth. The upper palatal cusps occlude with the fossae of the lower teeth. In a so-called lingualised occlusion, the lower buccal cusps are cut back so that there is only contact on the upper palatal cusps. This scheme allows the ease of obtaining a balanced occlusion comparable with the use of zero cusped teeth, together with the advantage of retaining poterior tooth cusp form and therefore a pleasing appearance.

Clinical considerations relating to occlusion

Determining occlusal vertical dimension

As described above, determining an acceptable OVD can be difficult. As discussed, the clinician has, however, to register an OVD and pass that information to the technician. Experienced clinicians usually rely on a combination of methods at the registration.

Recording centric jaw relation

Centric jaw relationship is a reproducible position that is used to articulate edentulous casts. The artificial teeth are set so that maximum intercuspation occurs at this position. Centric occlusion for complete dentures is the same as IP.

Many different methods have been described for recording CR. They may be classified as static or functional (Table 12.2). Most methods are capable of giving accurate results but functional techniques such as 'chew-in' techniques are not commonly used. The most common is the use of interocclusal wax occlusal rims.

Selecting an articulator for complete denture prosthodontics

As discussed previously, an average value articulator can be used with good results. However, in order to produce dentures with a balanced occlusion/articulation that should need minimal adjustment at insertion, a semiadjustable articulator together with the use of a facebow, and lateral and protrusive transfer records, should be considered.

Table 12.2 Methods of recording centric jaw relation	
Static	Functional
• Wax occlusal rims • Extraoral tracing (gothic arch) technique • Intraoral tracing device	• Chew-in techniques • Swallowing techniques

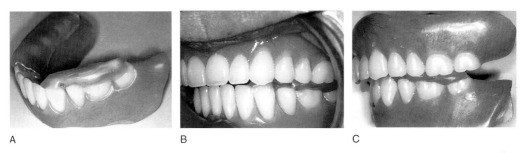

A   B   C

Fig. 12.3 Precentric check record. **A** Softened wax on the posterior mandibular teeth. **B** Patient has closed into the wax in the retruded arc of closure. Closing has stopped before the artificial teeth contact. **C** Precentric record removed from the mouth.

Setting up complete dentures

Setting of teeth requires considerable skill. The determinants of a balanced occlusion have been described above. Setting procedures for artificial teeth have been described in detail elsewhere (Zarb et al 1990).

Split-cast technique

As the acrylic resin cures during the processing of complete dentures, the artificial teeth can move slightly in the moulds. A split-cast technique is recommended to relocate complete dentures on the articulator following processing. This allows any minor occlusal errors that have occurred during processing to be corrected.

Occlusal correction at insertion

There are often occlusal interferences at the insertion stage as a result of inaccuracy of recording CR and limitations imposed by the articulator. Three methods are used to correct the occlusion: selective grinding, precentric (check) record and rerecording CR.

Selective grinding Minor errors are commonly detected with the use of articulating foil and corrected at the chairside. Because of the inherent instability of the denture bases, caution must be used when interpreting the marks made by the paper. Some clinicians consider that any adjustments should only be made with the use of a precentric (check) record, as described below.

There are two stages to chairside occlusal adjustment:

- The first objective is to ensure MI occurs in CR. Two possible errors may be present. One error occurs when the cusp–fossa relationships are correct but one or more teeth meet prematurely. To correct this type of error, the opposing fossae should be deepened until there is even bilateral contact. The other error is when there is misalignment of cusp–fossa relationships. This is corrected by first grinding mesial and distal slopes of opposing teeth, until cusp–fossa realignment is regained. The opposing fossae can then be deepened until even contact is established.

- The second objective of occlusal adjustment is to obtain a balanced occlusion. To readily achieve this the BULL (buccal upper, lingual lower) rule is recommended. It is the contacting surfaces of these cusps (the palatal surface of the upper buccal cusps and the buccal surfaces of the lower lingual cusps) that are ground, rather than the cusp tips.

If there is misalignment of cusp–fossa relationships, the cusps and their opposing embrasures should be adjusted by grinding mesial and distal cusp slopes of opposing teeth. The adjustment process should be continued until balanced occlusion is achieved.

Precentric (check) record More extensive errors can be eliminated using a precentric record. To do this, two layers of warm softened baseplate wax are placed on the lower premolars and molars. The patient is instructed/guided to close into the wax (but not to close into tooth contact) in the retruded position. The dentures are then articulated using this record and any errors are removed (Fig. 12.3). When the dentures are inserted, minor errors can be readily corrected as described.

Rerecording CR Occasionally the occlusal errors may be so large that chairside adjustment or even a check record could not correct the problem. In these cases, if the appearance of the anterior teeth is satisfactory, the posterior teeth should be ground off, wax can be placed on the base in those regions and CR can be rerecorded. The dentures can then be rearticulated, teeth reset and a denture try-in is repeated.

References

Palla S 1997 Occlusal considerations in complete dentures. In: McNeil C (ed) Science and practice of occlusion, Quintessence, Chicago, pp 457–467

Zarb G A, Bolender C L, Hickey J C, Carlsson G E (eds) 1990 Boucher's prosthodontic treatment for edentulous patients, 10th edn. Mosby, St Louis

Further reading

Dixon D L 2000 Overview of articulation materials and methods for the prosthodontic patient. Journal of Prosthetic Dentistry 235–247

Fenlon M R, Sherriff M, Walter J D 1999 Association between the accuracy of intermaxillary relations and complete denture usage. Journal of Prosthetic Dentistry 81: 520–525

Freilich M A, Altieri J V, Wahle J J 1992 Principles for selecting interocclusal records for articulation of dentate and partially dentate casts. Journal of Prosthetic Dentistry 68: 361–367

Murray M C, Smith P W, Watts D C, Wilson N G F 1999 Occlusal registration: science or art? International Dental Journal 49: 41–46

Rahn A O, Heartwell C M 1993 Relating inclinations of teeth to concepts of occlusion. In: Textbook of complete dentures, 5th edn. Lea & Febiger, Philadelphia, pp 357–371

Zarb G A, Bergman B, Clayton J A, MacKay H F (eds) 1978 Prosthodontic treatment for partially edentulous patients. Mosby, St Louis

13 Occlusion and implant restoration

J. Hobkirk

Synopsis

Dental implant occlusion has characteristics inherently similar to the natural and restored dentitions, and should be designed to mimic nature rather than create a purely mechanical system. Its design must therefore follow similar principles. These need to be modified to allow for the different characteristics of the support mechanism, and relate largely to the avoidance of mechanical overload of the patient–implant interface, the implant connecting components and the prosthetic superstructure.

The clinician has freedom to position implants in the most suitable locations, and these should be selected to minimise non-axial loads on the implants and reduce torquing as a result of cantilevering of the superstructure. This can occur both buccally and distally.

The occlusal scheme in the partially dentate patient should normally be conformative, and avoid localised stress concentration, for example by canine guidance. Where the full arch is reconstructed, then so-called 'balanced articulation' is preferred. Shallow cusp angles are associated with reduced implant loading.

There is little justification for using polymeric occlusal materials solely to minimise loads on implants. Ceramics or gold alloys perform better, but there may be aesthetic or technical limitations on their use, especially in larger constructions, when a resin-based aesthetic material may be preferred.

Implant occlusion should be designed during treatment planning, prior to implant placement. It involves implant location and superstructure design, as well as occlusal configuration, and is inherent in the treatment process.

Key points

- Implant occlusion is inherently similar to the occlusion of any other dental prosthesis. Its design relates not only to the occlusal surface, but also to its supporting mechanisms
- Objectives in occlusal design
  - Maximise occlusal function
  - Minimise harm to opposing and adjacent teeth
  - Minimise wear of occlusal surfaces
  - Minimise the risk of fracture of the implant superstructure
  - Reduce the risk of fracture of the implant body and its connecting components
  - Protect the implant–host interface; currently this is synonymous with maintaining osseointegration
- Particular characteristics of implant occlusion
  - Location: freedom potentially to locate implants in optimum locations
  - Displacability: an osseointegrated implant is displaced very little under load and behaves elastically
  - Immovability: implants cannot be moved by orthodontic forces
  - Proprioception: proprioceptive feedback is reduced
  - Force transmission: high forces may be generated by a patient with an implant-stabilised fixed bridge
  - Biomechanical overload: this is thought to be a key factor in the loss of osseointegration
  - Mechanical linkages: almost all dental implants employ mechanical linkages, many of which are prone to failure due to overload
- Force management is principally through the following design features:
  - implant location
  - occlusal form and scheme
  - superstructure design

EVIDENCE FROM THE LITERATURE

Early studies on dental implant occlusion centred on measurements of masticatory forces and occlusal tactile sensibility. While some of these used force transducers placed between the teeth, and were thus of little value in measuring functional loads, later studies using miniature intraoral transducers were able to demonstrate these. Such investigations showed that patients could generate higher occlusal forces with implant bridges than with conventional removable prostheses. It was also shown that they had a greater ability to detect thin films held between the teeth. Such investigations were intended to show the enhanced performance of implant bridges.

Subsequently it became evident that excessive occlusal forces could result in breakdown of the osseointegrated interface, although, apart from case reports, this work has been based on animal studies, with all the problems of their extrapolation to clinical practice. These findings lead to an increased interest in the potentially harmful effects of excessive loads, particularly since meta-analysis had demonstrated that mechanical failure of the implant and its superstructure was a major cause of problems once osseointegration had been achieved. Such studies were beset by the problem of defining and predicting an excessive load, however this is probably not solely limited to magnitude; frequency, load rate and duration may all be important, as is thought to be the structure of the bone itself. Currently we are lacking any clinically valid engineering data that would enable the predictive modelling of bone behaviour and facilitate implant selection, optimal placement and superstructure design.

Studies of shimstock perception lead to investigations into the phenomenon of osseoperception. These showed that patients with osseointegrated implants were able to detect applied forces, and that this changed with time. The exact mechanism is unknown, but is likely to involve nerve endings in the periosteum and mucosa, as well as those associated with the temporomandibular joints and muscles of mastication. Currently we lack detailed knowledge of this phenomenon and its potential diagnostic value.

Once there was awareness of the potential affects of force on osseointegration, both occlusal material and form came under scrutiny. It was postulated that acrylic resin would provide a shock-absorbing layer as compared with porcelain; however, while this could be demonstrated in vitro, it has never been shown clinically in a controlled manner. Studies on the effects of occlusal material on masticatory force have failed to demonstrate a linkage, as any possible effects are masked by the large variations between subjects and the moderating influence of the food being masticated.

Similarly, studies on occlusal form have tended to be carried out in vitro or in experimental animals, techniques that do not readily translate to the clinical scenario. They do, however, suggest that shallow cusp angles are favourable, and that bilateral occlusal contacts in lateral excursions of the mandible should be used with large constructions. Nevertheless, there is much advice on occlusal forms and schemes in implant prostheses, that has little if any clinical research base.

Studies of implant biomechanics lend themselves to physical investigations and modelling techniques, and there have been many such investigations using mechanical or computer-based methods of investigation. While helpful, they lack clinical veracity, a further area where much advice is empirical.

CLINICAL PRACTICE

Restorative dentistry is concerned with optimising oral function in terms of appearance, speech and mastication. This often, but not inevitably, requires the replacement of missing teeth and their supporting structures. Traditionally the partially dentate were treated with either fixed restorations or removable prostheses. The former were stabilised by linking them to the teeth using cemented joints on tapered tooth preparations, the latter with moveable joints based on clasps or precision attachments. Where lack of a suitable dentition or resources made this impossible, recourse had to be made to the alveolar ridges and the vertical surfaces of the teeth, employing the rather tenuous physical forces of friction, adhesion and cohesion. Apart from oral manipulative skills, only the latter two were available to the user of complete dentures.

The development of reliable implant techniques enabled these to be used as a third dentition, and they are now employed to stabilise single crowns, fixed bridges, removable partial dentures and complete overdentures. Restorative dentists have tended to carry over into implant dentistry the precepts and beliefs which sustained them when using these restorative techniques in the natural dentition, often with little justification. This applies equally to the design of the occlusion.

While it may be thought that there are quite enough approaches to this topic without adding another layer of complexity, nevertheless, the host–implant interface, and freedom to potentially locate implants at will, subject to anatomical constraints, create a different milieu.

What is implant occlusion?

In approaching this problem it is necessary to appreciate that we are concerned not solely with the shaping of the

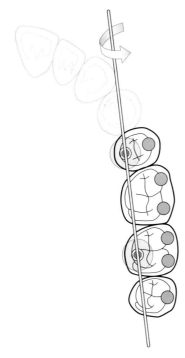

Fig. 13.1 Where implants supporting a fixed bridge lie palatal or lingual to the occlusal platform, then vertical forces on the teeth will tend to rotate the bridge around its fixing points on the implants.

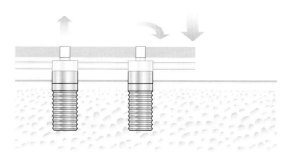

Fig. 13.2 Cantilevered occlusal surfaces result in rotational forces when loaded distally.

occlusal surfaces but more importantly with their location, extent and support. These factors will influence both function and, potentially, the integrity of the reconstruction itself, which extends from the bone around the implant to the load-receiving component of the system, the occlusal surface.

For the sake of simplicity the occlusal scheme provided for an implant-stabilised prosthesis is described here as an implant occlusion, that is, an occlusal scheme where a component of the forces applied to the dental prosthesis is transmitted to the orofacial skeleton by a dental implant.

While implant occlusion has similar requirements to that provided by a natural dentition, or one restored by other means, there are also requirements specific to such a situation. Our aims in designing an implant occlusion are to:

- maximise occlusal function
- minimise harm to opposing and adjacent teeth
- minimise wear of occlusal surfaces
- minimise the risk of fracture of the implant superstructure
- reduce the risk of fracture of the implant body and its connecting components

- protect the implant–host interface; currently this is synonymous with maintaining osseointegration.

If we are to achieve these aims then it is necessary to recognise the differences between tooth and implant-stabilised prostheses, and their significance for implant occlusion. Principally these are:

- *Location.* Freedom to potentially locate implants in optimum locations. Unfortunately this is often an illusory freedom due to anatomical constraints. A favourable relationship between an implant super-structure and its supporting implants can result in their being loaded optimally down their long axes, with torquing forces minimised. Where the relationship between the occlusal table and the implants is less suitable, then large torquing forces can arise as a result of implant orientation in available bone (e.g. the anterior maxilla), and buccal and distal cantilevering. The latter may also result in extraction forces on implants (Figs 13.1 and 13.2).
- *Rigidity under load.* An osseointegrated implant is displaced very little under load compared with a tooth. Osseointegrated implants also move in an essentially linear fashion under load, while teeth and soft tissues move in a viscoelastic manner. Consequently, if an occlusion made up of tooth- and implant-stabilised components has evenly distributed initial contacts in the intercuspal position (ICP), then after repeated loading the implant-supported contacts will be higher than those that are tooth-supported.
- *Immovability.* Implants cannot be moved by orthodontic forces. Occlusal modification by intrusion of an implant is not therefore feasible.
- *Proprioception.* Implants lack a periodontal membrane, and, it is thought, conventional proprioceptive feed-back. There is some evidence for perception related to implants, but it is ill understood and less sensitive than that of a natural tooth.

- *Force transmission.* Considerably higher forces may be generated by a patient with an implant-stabilised fixed bridge than with a conventional denture. This can result in apparent looseness of the opposing prosthesis and damage to the underlying tissues as a result of mechanical overload.
- *Biomechanical overload.* This is thought to be a key factor in the loss of osseointegration, which equates to implant failure. It is considered that transverse loads on dental implants are especially damaging. Values for potentially harmful forces are not known, and may be related not only to their magnitude, but also load rates and frequency. They may also be dependent on personal variation, bone quality, volume and shape, implant design and length, and superstructure design.
- *Mechanical linkages.* All dental implants employ mechanical linkages, of which screwed joints are the most common. These behave differently under load to the cemented or adhesive joints normally used in restorative dentistry. In particular, overload can result in their failure. While this characteristic is shared with restorations linked to natural teeth, the small size and mechanical complexity of dental implants makes fracture of implant superstructures and their retaining screws a common problem. The absence of engineering data for applied loads makes construction an empirical exercise. Undersized components, casting or soldering faults, excessive cantilevering and inappropriate occlusal schemes all increase the risk of failure.

These factors have considerable significance when designing an occlusal scheme for an implant superstructure, the principal function of which is to transmit occlusal forces to the facial skeleton. Where these are excessive in terms of magnitude, frequency or direction, damage to the prosthesis, implant or supporting tissues may ensue. Similarly, occlusal schemes which are not in harmony with their biological environment can give rise to problems, in the same fashion as those stabilised by underlying mucosa or abutment teeth. The principles that apply to these are no different and are described elsewhere in this book (Chs 1, 11 and 12).

The design of implant occlusion thus hinges around the creation of a functionally effective masticatory scheme that minimises occlusal loads, especially where they are not axial to the implant.

Force management

Given that it is not easy to measure functional occlusal loads clinically or to predict their effects, the clinician must rely on conventional wisdom for guidance. This suggests that:

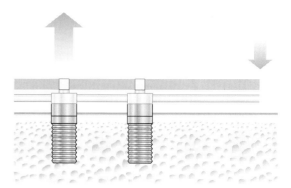

Fig. 13.3 Loads on a distal cantilever are magnified by leverage effects.

- Occlusal forces should be axially directed along the length of the implant.
- In a dentition restored with teeth and implants, initial occlusal contacts in ICP should occur only on the natural teeth.
- No clinical benefit has yet been shown for a particular occlusal surface material from the viewpoint of implant failure.
- Tipping forces on implants are harmful. These can arise as a result of cusp angulation, during lateral excursions of the mandible, and most significantly due to cantilevering of the superstructure (Fig. 13.3). This can be both distal and buccal, due to attempts to replace posterior teeth, or the need to place maxillary teeth lateral to the residual alveolar ridge in order to provide a natural appearance and normal relationship with the opposing teeth.
- Cyclical loads are more destructive because mechanical components are prone to fatigue failure.
- Loads on implants in the period after placement and when first loaded should be minimised. This reduces the risk of integration failing to occur due to excessive movement of the implant, or being lost in its early stages before it has matured.
- Implant treatment should be used with caution in patients with a bruxing habit.

DESIGNING THE OCCLUSION

Load management is an important dimension of occlusal design in implant treatment, as the scheme chosen will profoundly influence the forces that are generated. It covers implant location, extent and design of the occlusal surfaces, surface material, nature of the opposing dentition, and the type of superstructure.

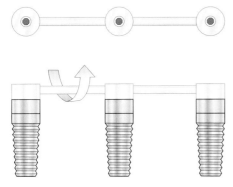

Fig. 13.4 A linear arrangement of dental implants provides little resistance to rotational forces.

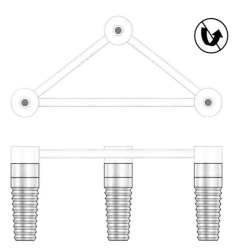

Fig. 13.5 A triangular orientation of implants, so called tripodisation, will effectively resist rotational forces.

Implant location

Masticatory forces are largely vertical to the occlusal plane, and higher in the molar region. They also have significant lateral components related to chewing patterns and cuspal angles. Lateral forces will tend to torque implants around their apical ends, and are thought to be more harmful to the bone–implant interface than vertical forces. They can also arise as a result of cantilevering of the superstructure both distally and buccally. The extent to which this arises will depend on whether a fixed or removable superstructure is employed. In the latter situation the linkage between the implant and the prosthesis may permit relative rotation, which will minimise torquing. Where implants are linked, horizontal forces will be more widely distributed and torquing reduced, especially if three or more implants are linked in a tripod fashion, as opposed to linearly. (Figs 13.4 and 13.5).

A further effect of cantilevering is to magnify and reverse the direction of occlusal forces due to leverage effects; it is for this reason that cantilever lengths are recommended to be typically 10 mm and no more than 15 mm.

Occlusal form and scheme

While extensive research on the effects of occlusal design on the outcome of implant treatment is limited, a number of general principles are emerging on the basis of a small number of studies and clinical experience.

Where a single implant is to be restored, or a small implant bridge provided, the occlusal scheme should be conformative. Group function is to be preferred to canine guidance, which should be avoided on an implant superstructure as the high local forces can lead to fracture of the crown, linking components or even the implant.

Where a full arch construction is utilised then 'balanced articulation' should be provided in order to minimise local loading and maximise stability of the prosthesis. There is some evidence that a degree of horizontal freedom of movement in ICP is helpful, while in vitro studies have shown that shallow cusp angles may be associated with reduced horizontal loading of an implant during mastication.

Occlusal contacts on implant superstructures, which are above the level of the adjacent teeth by 100–250 µm, have been shown in experimental animals to have a negative effect on bone formation adjacent to the implant in the crestal region. Studies on occlusal forces have also shown that loads on cantilevered implant superstructures are reduced significantly when their occlusal surfaces are slightly below those of adjacent teeth, whether natural or implant-stabilised.

Occlusal material

The preferred material for the occlusal surface of implant superstructures is still debated. At one time it was believed that acrylic resin would cushion occlusal loads to the benefit of the osseointegrated interface; however, this energy absorbing effect appears to be minimal compared with that of the food and individual variation in occlusal forces. In these circumstances, other factors need to be considered, such as longevity, abrasion resistance, appearance, ease of fabrication and ease of repair.

Acrylic or other resins, especially those with inorganic fillers, are often used for their ease of manipulation and flexibility. They also are less prone to mechanical failure in bulk, which can be a problem with extensive porcelain-faced metal frameworks. Such polymeric materials have poor wear resistance, and it is not uncommon for them to need replacement after 1–3 years, or even less when opposed by a natural dentition, especially if masticatory forces are high. Where this is a problem, gold alloy occlusal surfaces can provide an effective solution in both extensive fixed restorations and implant-stabilised complete dentures, although their appearance is not acceptable to all patients.

The design of the occlusion for implant prostheses is an integral part of treatment planning and should begin prior to implant insertion. It involves consideration of the occlusal scheme, the extent of the occlusal platform, implant location, control of horizontal forces, the achievement of axial implant loading where possible, implant location and the optimisation of appearance. Unfortunately it is often an afterthought, attempted with articulating paper and a handpiece, resulting in a suboptimal outcome.

Further reading

Denissen H W, Kalk W, van Wass M A J, van Os J H 1993 Occlusion for maxillary dentures opposing osseointegrated mandibular prostheses. International Journal of Prosthodontics 6:446–450

De Pauw G A, Dermaut L, De Bruyn H, Johansson C 1999 Stability of implants as anchorage for orthopedic traction. Angle Orthodontist 69(5):401–407

Duyck J, Van Oosterwyck H, Vander Sloten J et al 2000 Magnitude and distribution of occlusal forces on oral implants supporting fixed prostheses: an in vivo study. Clinical Oral Implants Research 11(5):465–475

Duyck J, Ronold H J, Van Oosterwyck H et al 2001 The influence of static and dynamic loading on marginal bone reactions around osseointegrated implants: an animal experimental study. Clinical Oral Implants Research 12(3):207–218

Kaukinen J A, Edge M J, Lang B R 1966 The influence of occlusal design on simulated masticatory forces transferred to implant-retained prostheses and supporting bone. Journal of Prosthetic Dentistry 76:50–55

Klineberg I, Murray G 1999 Osseoperception: sensory function and proprioception. Advances in Dental Research 130:120–129

Miyata T, Kobayashi Y, Araki H, Ohto T, Shin K 2000 The influence of controlled overload on peri-implant tissue. Part 3: A histologic study in monkeys. International Journal of Oral and Maxillofacial Implants 15(3):425–431

Richter E-J 1998 In vivo horizontal bending moments on implants. International Journal of Oral and Maxillofacial Implants 13:232–244

Stanford C M, Brand R A 1999 Towards an understanding of implant occlusion and strain adaptive bone modelling and remodelling. Journal of Prosthetic Dentistry 81(5):553–561

Van Steenberghe D, Naert I, Jacobs R, Quirynen M 1999 Influence of inflammatory reactions vs. occlusal loading on peri-implant marginal bone level. Advances in Dental Research 13:130–135

Weinberg L A 2001 Therapeutic biomechanics concepts and clinical procedures to reduce implant loading. Part I. Journal of Oral Implantology 27(6):293–301

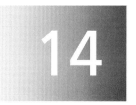

14 Occlusal splints and management of the occlusion

T. Wilkinson

Synopsis

Occlusal splints have been used for more than a hundred years to manage jaw dysfunction and they continue to be a common treatment modality. Hypotheses have been suggested to explain their action, but lack scientific validation.

There is general agreement that splints protect against tooth wear, and are valuable in preparation for dental treatment especially with complex restorative procedures including change of occlusal vertical dimension or jaw position. However, it has been difficult to establish the efficacy of splints in the management of temporomandibular disorders (TMDs). Although many studies claim that splints reduce nocturnal bruxism, others have shown that this does not occur, and some patients show increased jaw muscle force while wearing a splint.

The use of better study design in recent years has improved our understanding of splint efficacy. Pain reduction has been shown to occur in treatment and control groups, suggesting that this may be due to a placebo effect as well as the natural regression of symptoms with time. Stabilisation (or Michigan) splints and palatal splints (no occlusal coverage, used as a study control) were found to be more effective than using 'inactive control' splints (worn only during review visits) or 'no splint' control.

Trials have also shown that there was no apparent difference between a stabilisation splint and a non-occluding palatal appliance, suggesting that pain reduction is not due to a change in mandibular position or sensorimotor feedback, but to a non-specific behavioural response.

These recent reviews suggest that there is sufficient evidence to support the use of splints as adjuncts to treatment for localised myalgia or arthralgia. The most common design is the full upper arch, flat plane stabilisation (or Michigan) splint (Fig. 14.1).

This chapter details the clinical and laboratory stages of preparing this appliance and procedures for its adjustment and use.

Key points

- *Impression-taking*. The splint covers all teeth on the upper arch and opposes all lower teeth. Accurate alginate impressions of both arches are required, and these can be taken in stock trays
- *Transfer records*. A facebow may be used to transfer the relationship of the maxilla to the intercondylar axis and Frankfort horizontal. An interocclusal (or maxillomandibular, MMR) record records the relationship of the mandible to the maxilla in centric relation
- *Mounting casts on the articulator*. A semiadjustable articulator is suitable for splint construction and may be set to average condylar values. The maxillary cast is articulated using the facebow transfer, and the mandibular cast using the occlusal record
- *Block-out undercuts*. An ideal path of insertion is determined for the splint, and undesirable undercuts are blocked out
- *Splint fabrication*. Frictional retention is provided by the amount of buccal and labial tooth coverage. The flat occlusal table of the splint provides point contact for the buccal cusps of the lower molars and premolars. The tips of the canines and incisors contact a narrower anterior ledge. An anterior ramp provides guidance for canine or anterior teeth in lateral and protrusive movements

- *Intraoral adjustment*. Adjustment of the inner surface of the splint after processing may be required to provide a firm and comfortable fit. The occlusal table is adjusted to provide even and simultaneous bilateral contact in retruded contact position (RCP) and then to a 'long centric'. The anterior ramp is then adjusted to provide anterior guidance without molar contacts
- *Patient instructions*. Patients are instructed to use the splint while sleeping. Good oral hygiene needs to be emphasised and patients are instructed in the cleaning and storage of their splint
- *Review of splint*. Reviews are needed as part of a long-term management strategy. The splint may need to be adjusted if dental restorations are placed at a later time

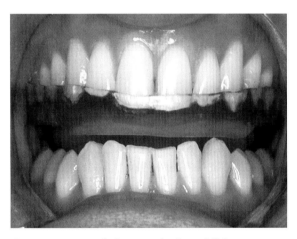

Fig. 14.1 Extraoral photograph of a stabilising (Michigan) splint seated on the maxillary teeth with the jaw slightly opened. Frictional retention is provided by 25% coverage of the labial surfaces of the incisors and canines, 33% coverage of the buccal surfaces of premolars and 50% coverage of the buccal surfaces of molars.

LITERATURE REVIEW

Early theories of the mode of action of splints were based on the concept that occlusal interferences caused masticatory muscle hyperactivity and parafunction, resulting in muscle pain and, in turn, increased hyperactivity (Travell & Rinzler 1952). This sequence of events was considered to be reduced or eliminated by the splint, as it provided an ideal occlusal scheme (Posselt 1968).

Laskin (1969) suggested that parafunction and the resultant pain and dysfunction were more related to the central effect of stress than to the peripheral role of occlusal irregularities. He described this condition as myofascial pain-dysfunction syndrome (MPD). This theory was reinforced by studies that showed a positive correlation between life events, nocturnal electromyographic (EMG) levels and masticatory muscle pain (Rugh & Solberg 1979).

Splints have been used to treat the less common muscle conditions described as myositis and myospasm, as well as the more common conditions described as myofascial pain and postexercise muscle soreness associated with bruxism. However, in recent years there has been controversy concerning the efficacy of occlusal splints in the treatment of TMDs. A National Institute of Health Conference in 1997, on the management of TMDs, reported that 'the efficacy of most treatment approaches for TMDs is unknown because most have not been adequately evaluated in long-term studies and virtually none in randomised controlled group trials. Moreover, their superiority to placebo controls or "no treatment" controls remains undetermined' (Lipton & Dionne 1997).

SPLINTS AND MUSCLE AND JOINT PAIN

Myofascial pain (fulfilling the Research Diagnostic Criteria for Temporomandibular Disorders (RDC/TMD) criteria of Dworkin and LeResche, 1992) has been reported in approximately 50% of patients presenting at a facial pain clinic (Fricton et al 1985). It is categorised by muscle tenderness, pain that can be made worse by function and referral of pain to other regions, and it is found in bruxing and non-bruxing patients. There is currently no convincing research-based evidence to explain the aetiology of myofascial pain.

Studies have shown the development of jaw muscle myalgia with voluntary clenching (Arima et al 1999). It has been suggested that subjects demonstrating intermittent bruxing at times of high stress may be exhibiting postexercise muscle soreness and that this is more likely to occur on waking. However, the majority of bruxers do not exhibit pain, and it has been suggested that their muscles may have adapted with time as a training effect. Studies of resting EMG levels in bruxers with pain were found to not be significantly different from bruxers without pain (Lund 2001). The poor correlation between pain and resting EMG contradicts the earlier 'vicious cycle' theory associated with occlusal irregularities.

Self-reports of pain among 19 confirmed nocturnal bruxers in a polysomnographic study were compared with 61 patients in another study with jaw muscle myofascial pain (RDC/TMD criteria) with no evidence of bruxism (Dao et al 1994a). Only six of the 19 bruxers experienced pain, and this typically occurred in the morning, whereas the majority of the myofascial group reported pain in the evening. The authors suggested that bruxism and jaw muscle myofascial pain might be distinct entities with different aetiologies.

Patients with treated splints for jaw muscle pain may have myositis myospasm conditions, myofascial pain or postexercise muscle soreness. Research evidence is lacking to determine whether these are discrete conditions; their aetiology and natural history and the role of bruxism is unclear. There may also be other conditions causing pain that have not yet been identified.

Occlusal splints have been shown to reduce nocturnal EMG levels, but their effect is variable and, in some studies, subjects have shown increases in activity. Clark (1988) reviewed the efficacy of these appliances and concluded that a strong association had been demonstrated between muscle hyperactivity and the symptoms of jaw pain, and that occlusal splints had been used effectively to treat this condition. However, the evidence is weak and care must be taken in drawing the conclusion that there is a cause and effect relationship between bruxism and the subgroups of TMDs.

Clark also reported on several theories proposed to explain how splints reduce symptoms (Clark 1988), including the provision of an interference-free occlusal scheme, alteration of vertical dimension, correction of the occlusion to centric relation, realignment of the TM joints and increased cognitive awareness. Dao and Lavigne (1998) reviewed these theories and concluded that the quality of the evidence was questionable and was based on unsubstantiated aetiologies.

The best evidence of therapeutic efficacy comes from systematic reviews of well-designed randomised controlled trials (RCTs). The incorporation of a control group is essential, as TMD symptoms fluctuate, there is a high rate of spontaneous remission and placebo effects may significantly contribute to symptom relief. Random assignment of patients to groups, and blinded data collection and analysis are essential to limit bias. The majority of past studies do not fulfil these requirements, and hence the true therapeutic value of splint therapy has not been established.

Dao et al (1994a) completed an RCT with 61 patients with myofascial pain (RDC/TMD criteria), divided into three groups: a treatment group, using a stabilisation (Michigan) splint 24 hours a day; a passive control group who wore a similar splint but only for 30 minutes at each review appointment; and an active control group who used a non-occluding palatal splint 24 hours a day. The patients' report of pain using a visual analogue scale (VAS) reduced significantly with time for all three groups and there was no significant difference between groups. They concluded that this study cast doubts on the therapeutic value of occlusal splints, and felt that the reduction in pain may have been due to placebo effects or spontaneous remission. This study caused considerable concern among clinicians, particularly as the results were thought to apply to jaw muscle pain in general.

However, the authors failed to indicate that they excluded patients with a history of bruxism. This only became evident when these same patients were reviewed in a subsequent paper (Dao et al 1994b). Hence the conclusions of the 1994 study for treatment efficacy are only valid for the TMD subgroup of myofascial pain without bruxism.

The outcome of the 1994 study was further analysed by the authors, who compared patients' reports at each visit of 'pain' (efficacy) with reports of 'pain relief' (effectiveness) (Feine et al 1995). They reported that 'pain relief' scores increased with time for each of the three groups but increased significantly less for the passive control group. They hypothesised that patients in the passive control group may have been increasingly convinced that they had not received 'true' treatment, which may have explained why they perceived treatment as being less efficacious. It is interesting to consider that patient satisfaction with treatment depends on factors other than pain relief. It would seem that there may have been differences in the strength of the placebo effect between groups, but this only became obvious when the outcome variable was changed from 'pain' to 'pain relief'. The authors concluded that, until the cause of TMDs is known, it was justifiable to provide a treatment that does not necessarily reduce pain but makes the patient feel better.

Ekberg et al (1998) carried out a similar RCT with a patient group with arthralgia (RDC/TMD criteria) and compared the efficacy of a stabilisation (Michigan) splint with a non-occluding but active palatal splint. Patients were not excluded because of a history of bruxism. VAS scores were used to assess pain intensity and no statistically significant differences were found between the stabilisation and palatal splint. However, when the outcome measure of 'perceived relief' was considered, the stabilisation splint was statistically superior to the palatal splint. This disagreed with the original study of Dao et al (Dao et al 1994a), but the authors considered that this was because the study was of patients with arthrogenous pain, whereas Dao's group studied patients with myofascial pain.

Several studies over the last 5 years have evaluated (meta-analyses) RCTs of splint therapy. Raphael and Marbach (1997) reviewed the literature on occlusal appliances for TMDs and reported that 'most controlled studies conclude that appliances are not effective'.

Dao and Lavigne (1998) reviewed similar literature and concluded that the true efficacy of splints is still questionable and that the improvement in pain in most studies may be due to non-specific effects of treatment such as placebo or regression to the mean. They considered that splints might have a place in changing harmful habits and promoting patients' perception of well-being. They concluded that until the natural history and aetiology of the different TMDs are determined and more specific treatment regimens are developed for these conditions, splints should only be used as an adjunct to pain management.

Forssell et al (1999) carried out a meta-analysis of RCTs of splint therapy and reported that the stabilisation splint was found to be superior to three, and comparable to 12, control treatments, and superior or comparable to four passive controls but expressed concern that palatal splints, acupuncture, ultrasound and TENS (transcutaneous electrical nerve stimulation) had been used as controls when these may have affected muscle function and the subject's cognitive awareness. They concluded that 'occlusal splints may be of benefit in the treatment of TMDs'.

Kriener et al (2001) reviewed RCTs of splint therapy. They suggested that differences in the TMD population studied may affect outcomes, with some studies only including myofascial pain patients and others including myogenous and arthrogenous subjects, and outcomes might vary between bruxer and non-bruxer populations.

They concluded that splints were operating in a similar way to the behavioural interventions of biofeedback and relaxation, and not as a medical device that was producing effects through physical changes in the position of the mandible. They felt that there was sufficient evidence to support the use of splints for the management of localised myalgia or arthralgia.

SPLINT CONSTRUCTION

Splint design

Design preferences vary widely between clinicians, who may choose upper or lower appliances, interlocking versus flat plane appliances, appliances with or without anterior guidance, and appliances of various thickness, but these preferences are not supported by outcome studies involving RCTs.

There may be differences in the choice of materials between hard versus soft appliances. Soft appliances may be preferred by clinicians because of their perceived comfort and for their ease of fitting. However, there is evidence to suggest that soft appliances are less effective in reducing bruxism (Kuboki et al 1997).

The most common appliance used around the world is the stabilisation (Michigan) splint. This is a rigid upper appliance with a flat occlusal plane and a ramp providing anterior guidance. It is usually constructed with minimal increase in vertical dimension consistent with providing strength, and is adjusted to even contact of all lower teeth in RCP or centric relation. This is the design that will be described in this text (Fig. 14.1).

Preparation of casts

Upper and lower alginate impressions in stock trays provide suitable casts in dental stone for splint construction.

A facebow may be used to transfer the relationship of the maxilla to the intercondylar axis and Frankfort horizontal; a maxillomandibular record is used to record the relationship of the maxillary and mandibular arches to complete the transfer record (Chs 1 and 6).

Frictional retention for the splint is provided by 25% coverage of the labial surfaces of the incisors and canines, 33% coverage of the buccal surfaces of premolars and 50% coverage of the buccal surfaces of molars (Fig. 14.1). It is important to block out undercuts on maxillary casts to reduce chairside time when fitting the appliance (Fig. 14.2). The appliance extends 5–10 mm into the palate beyond the palatal gingival margin.

Splint fabrication

A 2 mm thick thermosetting blank may be heated and pressure-moulded over the upper cast. Autopolymerising resin is adapted over the blank, and the articulator is then closed to determine the vertical dimension of the splint. The resin is shaped to provide a flat occlusal plane approximately 5 mm in width to be contacted by the buccal cusps of the lower molar and premolar teeth (Fig. 14.3). The canine and incisor teeth contact a narrower 2 mm flat anterior ledge. An anterior ramp with a 45° slope extends from this ledge to provide guidance in

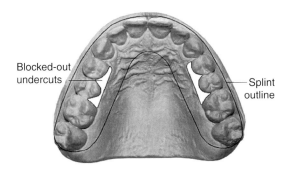

Blocked-out undercuts

Splint outline

Fig. 14.2 The outline of splint extensions and lingual undercuts blocked out with plaster.

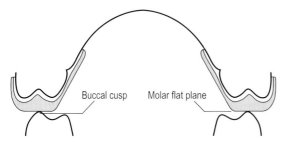

Fig. 14.3 A frontal section through the upper first molars showing a 2 mm thermosetting blank adapted over the molar surface and palate. The acrylic addition provides a flat plane against which the buccal cusp of the lower molars occludes.

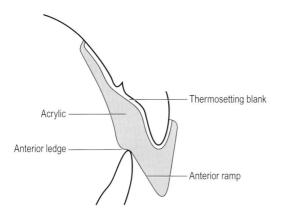

Fig. 14.4 A sagittal section through an upper central incisor showing a 2 mm thermosetting blank adapted over the upper incisor and palate with acrylic resin build-up to provide an anterior ledge and a 45° anterior ramp.

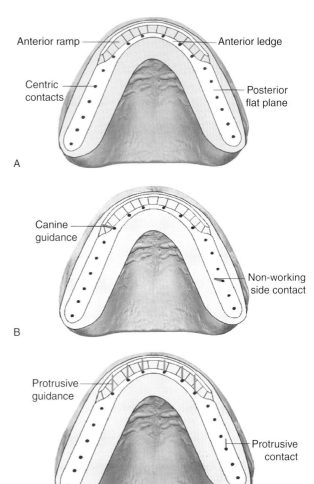

Fig. 14.5 An occlusal splint. **A** A horizontal flat plane (white) contacted by the buccal cusps of the lower molar and premolars and the narrower horizontal anterior ledge (white) contacted by the lower canines and incisors. The 45° anterior ramp (grey) arises immediately from the point of contact of the lower anterior teeth. **B** The laterotrusive path of the lower right canine tooth against the anterior ramp during a right-sided lateral excursion. The mediotrusive path of the lower left first molar is shown as a non-working side contact. **C** The path of the lower incisor and canine teeth against the anterior ramp during a protrusive movement. The path of the lower left first molar is shown as a protrusive contact.

lateral and protrusive mandibular movements (Fig. 14.4). The resin is then processed in a pressure flask to reduce porosity.

Laboratory splint adjustment

The splint is adjusted on the articulator, with plastic articulating tape, to provide simultaneous RCP contact of incisor and canine tips and premolar and molar buccal cusps in centric relation (Fig. 14.5A). These centric contacts are marked in one colour and the path of the tips of the lower teeth during lateral and protrusive excursions are marked against the anterior ramp in a different colour (Fig. 14.5B, C). The splint is adjusted so that the ipsilateral lower canine tip is the only tooth contacting during lateral excursion and the incisor and canine tips are the

only teeth contacting the splint in protrusion eliminating any contralateral or protrusive contacts on molars or premolars.

The splint is then removed from the cast and the palate removed. The labial, buccal and palatal extensions are

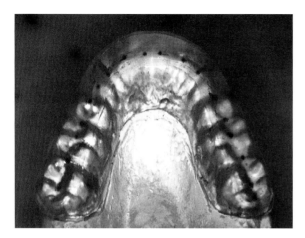

Fig. 14.6 An intraoral occlusal view of a stabilising (Michigan) splint showing a flat plane occlusal surface with an anterior ramp. Articulator tape markings show right and left canine guidance on the anterior ramp and the centric contacts of the lower teeth.

polished (Fig. 14.6). The occlusal surface is left unpolished so that articulating tape leaves clear marks during splint adjustment in the mouth.

Intraoral adjustment

Judicious blocking out of undercuts during construction reduces chairside time in fitting the splint. Pressure indicator paste may be used to disclose any points on the fitting surface that are preventing the splint from fully seating or causing rocking.

The occlusal surface of the splint is then adjusted to even and simultaneous contact of the tips of all lower anterior teeth and all buccal cusps of molar and premolar teeth in centric relation. Miller holders that support articulating paper assist these adjustments. Some clinicians may allow the patient 'freedom in centric' by adjusting the occlusal surface to even contact of lower teeth at median occlusal position (MOP) – a 'snap jaw closure' that brings the mandible slightly forward from RCP.

The anterior ramp is then adjusted to provide smooth incisal and canine guidance in lateral movement and incisal guidance during protrusion.

Patient instructions

Patients are instructed to use the appliance only during sleep. They are advised that some patients occasionally take splints out during sleep without waking, and that splints may increase or decrease salivation during sleep. They may find the splint may be tight on different teeth

from time to time but this discomfort will reduce with continued use. Patients are instructed to monitor their oral hygiene because of the risk of increased plaque accumulation around their teeth and inside the splint.

Review of splint

Review appointments assess that occlusal contacts on the splint are stable and are used to reinforce avoidance of daytime parafunction habits. Reviews every 2 months over the first 6 months are desirable to determine when symptoms improve, indicating that patients may start to reduce the frequency of splint wear. There may be a need to return to using the splint if symptoms worsen or if they realise from their self-monitoring that there has been an increase in clenching, particularly during stress.

Patients should be informed that teeth might move slightly if they cease using the splint for a period and that any initial discomfort or tightness will settle on resuming splint use. Patients using splints on a long-term basis should be reviewed every 12 months to ensure there is no occlusal or periodontal change. Splints may need to be adjusted after new restorations.

References

Arima T, Svensson P, Arendt-Nielsen L 1999 Experimental grinding in healthy subjects: a cast for postexercise jaw muscle soreness. Journal of Orofacial Pain 13:104–114

Clark G T 1988 Interocclusal appliance therapy. In: Mohl N D, Zarb G A, Carlsson G E, Rugh I D (eds) A textbook of occlusion. Quintessence, Chicago, pp 271–284

Dao T T, Lavigne G J 1998 Oral splints: the crutches for temporomandibular disorders and bruxism? Critical Reviews in Oral Biology and Medicine 9:345–361

Dao T T, Lavigne G J, Charonneau A, Feine J S, Lund J P 1994a The efficacy of oral splints in the treatment of myofascial pain of the jaw muscles; a controlled clinical trial. Pain 56:85–94

Dao T T, Lund J P, Lavigne G J 1994b Comparison of pain and quality of life in bruxers and patients with myofascial pain of the masticatory muscles. Journal of Orofacial Pain 8:350–355

Dworkin S F, LeResche L 1992 Research diagnostic criteria for temporomandibular disorders: review, criteria, examinations and critique. Journal of Craniomandibular Disorders: Facial and Oral Pain 6:301–355

Ekberg E C, Vallon D, Nilner M 1998 Occlusal appliance therapy in patients with temporomandibular disorders: a double-blind controlled study in a short-term perspective. Acta Odontologica Scandinavica 56:122–128

Feine J S, Lavigne G J, Lund J P 1995 Assessment of treatment efficacy for chronic orofacial pain. In: Morimoto T, Matsuya T, Takada K (eds) Brain and oral functions. Elsevier, Amsterdam, pp 257–264

Forssell H, Kalso E, Koskela P et al 1999 Occlusal treatments in temporomandibular disorders: a qualitative systematic review of randomised controlled trials. Pain 83:549–560

Fricton J R, Kroenig R, Haley D, Siegert R 1985 Myofascial pain syndrome to the head and neck: a review of clinical characteristics of 164 patients. Oral Surgery 60:615–623

Kriener M, Betancor E, Clark G T 2001 Occlusal stabilisation appliances: evidence of their efficacy. Journal of the American Dental Association 132:770–777

Kuboki T, Azuma Y, Orsini M et al 1997 The effect of occlusal appliances and clenching on the temporomandibular joint space. Journal of Orofacial Pain 11:67–77

Laskin D M 1969 Etiology of the pain-dysfunction syndrome. Journal of the American Dental Association 79:147–153

Lipton J A, Dionne R A 1997 National Institutes of Health technology assessment conference on management of temporomandibular disorders. Oral Surgery, Oral Medicine, Oral Pathology and Endodontics; 83:49–183

Lund J P 2001 Pain and movement. In: Lund J P, Lavigne G J, Dubner R, Sessle B J (eds) Orofacial pain: from basic science to clinical management. Quintessence, Chicago, pp 151–163

Posselt U 1968 Physiology of occlusion and rehabilitation, 2nd edn. F A Davis, Philadelphia

Raphael K, Marbach J J 1997 Evidence-based care of musculoskeletal facial pain. Implications for the clinical science of dentistry. Journal of the American Dental Association 128:73–79

Rugh J D, Solberg W K 1979 Psychological implications in temporomandibular pain and dysfunction. In: Zarb G A, Carlsson G E (eds) Temporomandibular joint function and dysfunction. Munksgaard, Copenhagen, pp 239–258

Travell J G, Rinzler S H 1952 The myofascial genesis of pain. Postgraduate Medicine 11:425–434

15

The role of occlusal adjustment

A. Au, I. Klineberg

Synopsis

Occlusal adjustment is important in prosthodontic pretreatment and has been used for selected cases of temporomandibular disorders (TMDs). The clinical procedure involves tooth surface reduction and tooth surface addition with an appropriate restorative material. Occlusal adjustment is distinguished from occlusal equilibration and selective grinding with clear indications and aims. A systematic preclinical and clinical approach has clear advantages for long-term stability of treatment. There is, however, disagreement regarding terminology and the scientific justification of this irreversible procedure in the management of TMDs and, in particular, chronic orofacial pain. This chapter aims to clarify definitions and examines research evidence available for the application of occlusal adjustment in the management of TMDs and chronic orofacial pain.

Key points

- Occlusal adjustment may involve tooth surface reduction and/or tooth surface addition
- Occlusal adjustment is different from occlusal equilibration and selective grinding
- Specific aims and indications are described for occlusal adjustment
- Occlusal adjustment should only be used where there is clear and justifiable indication
- There is no strong evidence to indicate that it is more effective than conservative reversible procedures in treatment of TMDs. Nor is there evidence for its use in the management of chronic orofacial pain

- It is recommended that occlusal adjustment be planned on articulated study casts before being attempted clinically
- The use of a vacuum-formed template allows accurate implementation of preplanned occlusal adjustment

INTRODUCTION

Occlusal adjustment is a procedure whereby selected areas of tooth surface, in dentate or partially dentate patients, are modified to provide improved tooth and jaw stability and to direct loading to appropriate teeth during lateral excursions. This may involve tooth surface reduction and tooth surface addition with a restorative material. Where tooth surface reduction is required, this is completed with minimal adjustment. There is evidence from case–control studies that reduction of tooth contact interferences may reduce specific signs and symptoms of TMDs, such as temporomandibular (TM) joint clicking (Pullinger et al 1993, Au et al 1994). However, these are not prospective controlled studies. Where tooth surface addition is required, a restorative material may be added to enhance buccolingual and mesiodistal stability of strategic teeth or to provide more definite guiding inclines for lateral guidance.

Occlusal adjustment is distinguished from occlusal equilibration and selective grinding.

Occlusal equilibration

This is carried out to produce a specific occlusal scheme, generally in severely debilitated dentitions, requiring extensive restorative treatment. It is usually designed to achieve:

- coincidence between retruded contact position (RCP) and intercuspal contact position (ICP)
- precise cusp to fossa or cusp to marginal ridge contacts

- anterior guidance resulting in disclusion of posterior teeth with lateral jaw movement.

Occlusal equilibration may require extensive tooth modification to develop the prescribed occlusal scheme. Those features may be achieved with fixed restorative procedures.

Selective grinding

This is the reshaping of one or more teeth to reduce or alter specific undesirable occlusal contacts or tooth inclinations. It may be carried out to reduce plunger cusps, over-erupted posterior teeth with unopposed contacts, wedging or locking effects of restorations or extruded teeth, each of which may prevent freedom of the jaw to move anteriorly and laterally without tooth contact interferences. Selective grinding has also been used as an adjunct treatment in different disciplines, including periodontics, orthodontics, general restorative dentistry and endodontics, but is often incorrectly termed 'occlusal adjustment' in the literature. The references listed under Further reading provide examples of its use in different dental disciplines.

Aims of occlusal adjustment

- To maintain intra-arch stability by providing an occlusal plane with minimal curvature anteroposteriorly and minimal lateral curve. This minimises the effect of tooth contact interferences.
- To maintain interarch stability by providing bilateral synchronous contacts on posterior teeth in RCP and ICP at the correct occlusal vertical dimension (OVD). Supporting cusps of posterior teeth are in a stable contact relationship with opposing fossae or marginal ridges.
- To provide guidance for lateral and protrusive jaw movements on mesially directed inclines of anterior teeth, or as far anteriorly as possible. Posterior guiding contacts are modified so as not to be a dominant influence in lateral jaw movements. This is a commonly accepted practice in developing a therapeutic occlusion as it is clinically convenient. However, there is inadequate evidence from controlled studies to justify its routine use in the natural dentition.
- To allow optimum disc–condyle function along the posterior slope of the eminence, by encouraging smooth translation and rotation of the condyle.
- To provide freedom of jaw movement anteriorly and laterally. This overcomes a restricted functional angle of occlusion (FAO) caused by in-locked tooth relationships. A restricted FAO arises in the following types of tooth arrangements: deep anterior overbite, undercontoured

restorations with loss of OVD, extruded teeth and plunger cusps. This has been a traditionally accepted practice in restorative dentistry. Although there appear to be subjective benefits for the patient, these are not verified by controlled clinical trials.

Indications for occlusal adjustment

- As a pretreatment in prosthodontics and general restorative care:
  - to improve jaw relationships and provide stable tooth contacts for jaw support in ICP
  - to improve the stability of individual teeth.
- To enhance function by providing smooth guidance for lateral and protrusive jaw movements. This may involve modification of plunger cusps, in-locked cuspal inclines and mediotrusive, laterotrusive and protrusive tooth contact interferences.
- To modify a traumatic occlusion where tooth contact interferences are associated with excessive tooth loading, such as may occur in parafunctional clenching, resulting in tooth sensitivity, abfractions or fractures and/or increased tooth mobility. Occlusal adjustment will direct loading to appropriate teeth in an optimal direction and where possible, along their long axes.
- To stabilise orthodontic, restorative or prosthodontic treatment. In such cases where it is decided that existing restorations are to be retained, an occlusal adjustment may be indicated. Alternatively, adjustment in conjunction with occlusal build-up on selected teeth may be required.

Occlusal adjustment has been used both as a pretreatment restorative procedure involving fixed and removable prosthodontics, and as adjunctive therapy in the treatment of TMDs. Improved neuromuscular harmony as well as signs and symptoms of TMDs following occlusal adjustment procedures have been described in a randomised controlled study by Forssell et al (1987), but the evidence is weakened by the presence of non-homogenous study groups and mixed therapies. The effect of occlusal adjustment on sleep bruxism has also been investigated in uncontrolled studies (Bailey & Rugh 1980). Clark et al (1999) reviewed articles that described the effect of experimentally induced occlusal interferences on healthy, non-TMD subjects. Symptoms including transient tooth pain and mobility were reported, and changes in postural muscle tension levels and disruption of smooth jaw movements were noted. Occasional jaw muscle pain and TM joint clicking were also observed. However, the data do not strongly support a link between experimentally induced occlusal interferences and TMDs. Tsukiyama et al (2001) provided a critical review of published data on occlusal adjustment as a treatment for TMDs and concluded that current evidence does not support the use of occlusal adjustment in preference to other conservative therapies in the treatment of bruxism and non-tooth-related TMDs. This is not surprising as there are no randomised controlled trials demonstrating a link between tooth contact interferences and aetiology of bruxism or chronic orofacial pain. There is some evidence that tooth contact interferences may be related to jaw muscle pain and TMDs by their effects on directional guidance of teeth in function. However, evidence from current studies is weak, as direct comparison between the studies is not possible due to:

- difference in philosophy between various researchers regarding mandibular/condylar position and the method of achieving RCP during occlusal adjustment
- difference in philosophy of the occlusal contact scheme
- lack of a standardised approach to the measurement of the study and outcome factors
- lack of clearly defined TMD diagnostic subgroups in treatment subjects
- lack of adequate blinding during the experiments
- small sample size with sometimes high subject loss to follow-up
- short follow-up periods
- non-standardised control treatments
- poorly defined study bases (hospital or pain clinic populations)
- no adjusting for potential confounders or effect modifiers.

If the efficacy of occlusal adjustment is to be demonstrated, well-designed multicentre studies using clearly defined diagnostic subgroups, with large sample sizes and long follow-up periods are necessary. Until then, the recommendations of the Neuroscience Group of the International Association for Dental Research, through its consensus statement on TMDs (2002), should be heeded: 'it is strongly recommended that, unless there are specific and justifiable indications to the contrary, treatment should be based on the use of conservative, reversible and preferably evidence-based therapeutic modalities. While no specific therapies have been proven to be uniformly effective, many of the conservative modalities have proven to be at least as effective in providing palliative relief as various forms of invasive treatment, and they present much less risk of producing harm'.

CLINICAL PRACTICE

Clinical occlusal adjustment is facilitated by carrying out the procedure initially on study casts, articulated on an adjustable articulator by accurate transfer records

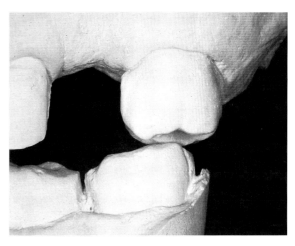

Fig. 15.1 Mediotrusive interference on the palatal cusp of the upper second molar demonstrated on articulated casts.

(Fig. 15.1). There are advantages in treatment planning in this way:

- Clinical time is reduced, as treatment planning decisions have been made concerning the optimum areas of tooth structure to be adjusted, following analysis and adjustment of study casts. It is then relatively easy to follow the pattern of adjustment determined on casts when completing an adjustment clinically.
- Diagnostic occlusal adjustment on articulated study casts also allows assessment of the amount of tooth surface reduction required. If the diagnostic adjustment indicates that removal of tooth structure is excessive, other forms of management such as tooth surface addition, orthodontic treatment or onlay-dentures may be considered.
- Areas of tooth adjustment are carefully selected, as failure to do so may undermine occlusal stability, leading to further deterioration of the existing disorder.

Equally important is the presentation of the diagnostic adjustment to the patient, illustrating the reason for the procedure and the teeth to be modified, to ensure that informed consent is obtained. This may be of importance in one's defence should a dentolegal problem arise. The following text describes an accurate method for transposing the preplanned occlusal adjustment, as already performed on articulated casts, to the correct areas of tooth structure in the mouth.

Preclinical preparation

The preclinical sequence to be followed includes verification of the articulation of casts when transfer

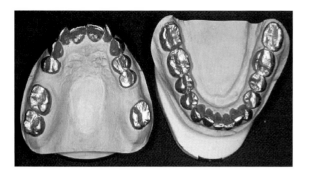

Fig. 15.2 The teeth of the upper and lower duplicate casts painted with die spacer in preparation for preclinical laboratory occlusal adjustment.

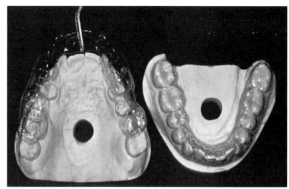

Fig. 15.3 Clear thermoplastic templates made over unadjusted casts. The centre vent hole in the casts allows improved adaptation of the thermoplastic material to the casts.

records are taken. Kerr occlusal indicator wax (Kerr, Emeryville, USA) is used to record RCP contacts. This record is chilled, removed from the mouth and taken to the laboratory, where the perforation points are checked against the initial contact points of the articulated casts. Coincidence of these indicates an accurate articulation of casts. Tru-fit dye spacer (George Taub Products and Fusion Co. Inc., Jersey City, USA) or a text highlighting pen with a different colour from the stone cast may be used to cover contacting surfaces of all upper and lower teeth (Fig. 15.2). The occlusal adjustment sequence is carried out on the articulated casts as follows:

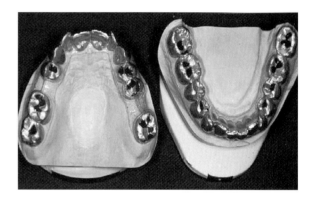

Fig. 15.4 Templates placed over adjusted duplicate casts. Adjusted areas are highlighted with ink to allow clear identification. Wax has been added to the palatal surface of tooth 13 to represent the area where composite resin will be placed to provide an occlusal contact.

- RCP contacts are adjusted to provide well-distributed bilateral synchronous contacts, providing optimum jaw support.
- ICP contacts are adjusted to provide well-distributed bilateral synchronous points of tooth contact.
- The slide between RCP and ICP will be reduced or eliminated; however, routine elimination of this slide is not an essential requirement.
- Mediotrusive interferences are eliminated to allow laterotrusive guidance on canines (canine guidance) or canines and bicuspids, or canines, bicuspids and molar teeth (group function).
- Laterotrusive adjustment is completed when it is possible to move the maxillary cast in a lateral and lateroprotrusive direction without interference, with the canines or canines in conjunction with posterior teeth providing guidance.
- Protrusive contacts are adjusted to allow canines and incisors to provide protrusive guidance. The adjustment is restricted to regions between cusps where possible. Care is taken to preserve supporting cusp tips and to recontour cuspal inclines, opposing fossae or marginal ridges, thus providing cusp tip to fossa or marginal ridge contacts.

Minimal tooth adjustment is emphasised and adjustments are confined where possible to the maxillary arch. The adjusted areas of the casts are then marked with ink to allow clear identification. A clear thermoplastic vacuum-formed template (Bego adaptor foils, 0.6 mm thickness) is drawn down over the original cast (Fig. 15.3) and then placed over the adjusted cast (Fig. 15.4). With the use of a sharp scalpel or a flat fissure burr, areas on the template corresponding to the adjusted areas on the cast are carefully removed. The template is trimmed (Fig. 15.5) around its entire periphery to restrict its extensions to only 2 mm beyond the gingival margins. The peripheries are smoothed to remove sharp edges that may traumatise intraoral soft tissues.

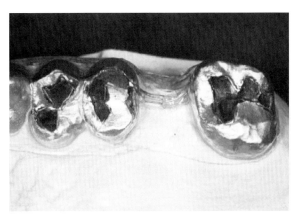

Fig. 15.5 Trimmed templates over adjusted casts (palatal view). Perforations in the template correspond to adjusted areas of tooth cusps on the cast.

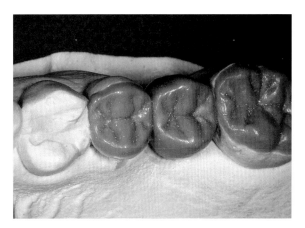

Fig. 15.7 Completed occlusal adjustment is shown; it is a preparatory step for three-unit bridgework in the upper posterior quadrants. Diagnostic wax-up of the planned restorations are made on study casts of the adjusted dentition. If no further treatment was required, adjusted tooth areas would be polished and fluoride applied to complete treatment.

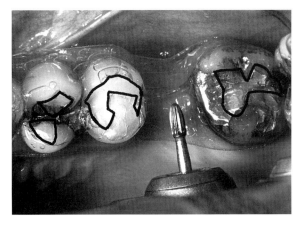

Fig. 15.6 Upper template in position on upper teeth. Areas of tooth to be adjusted protrude through the prepared template perforations and are indicated by the highlighted outlines.

Clinical procedures

The template is seated over the teeth and examined for accuracy of fit around the teeth. It should not cause discomfort to the soft tissues. The areas of tooth cusp or marginal ridge to be adjusted are clearly visible protruding through the prepared perforations of the template (Fig. 15.6). A pear-shaped composite finishing diamond (Komet 8368.204.016) or 12-fluted tungsten carbide burr (Komet H46.014) is recommended to adjust the teeth. Areas of tooth structure protruding beyond the perforations in the template are removed (Fig. 15.6). Where addition of a restorative material is required, a thermoplastic vacuum-formed template can be made over a duplicate of the

diagnostic wax-up. The template can be used clinically to assist the precise placement of composite resin in the prepared areas. This represents the initial adjustment stage.

The occlusal adjustment may then be refined and completed. The adjustments are checked repeatedly using plastic articulating tape (GHM foil – Gebr. Hansel-Medizinal, Nurtingen, Germany; Ivoclar/Vivadent, Schaan, Liechtenstein) as well as the clinician's tactile sense:

- RCP adjustment is checked to ensure well-distributed bilateral stops on supporting cusps.
- ICP adjustment is checked also for bilateral stops. This may eliminate or reduce the magnitude of an RCP/ICP slide.
- Mediotrusive interferences are refined to ensure canine or anterior guidance or group function in laterotrusion.
- Protrusive interferences are refined to allow guidance on canines or canine and incisor teeth.
- All adjusted tooth surfaces are polished and topical fluoride applied.
- Impressions of the adjusted teeth are taken and a diagnostic wax-up of planned restorations are made on articulated study casts of the adjusted occlusion (Fig. 15.7).

Acknowledgement

We would like to express our thanks to Mr Charles Kim for his preparation of the laboratory technical work.

References

Au A, Ho C, McNeil D W, Klineberg I 1994 Clinical occlusal evaluation of patients with craniomandibular disorders. Journal of Dental Research 73:739 (abstract)

Bailey J O, Rugh I D 1980 Effect of occlusal adjustment on bruxism as monitored by nocturnal EMG recordings. Journal of Dental Research 59:317 (abstract)

Clark G T, Tsukiyama Y, Baba K, Watanabe T 1999 Sixty-eight years of experimental occlusal interference studies: what have we learned? Journal of Prosthetic Dentistry 82:704–713

Forssell H, Kirveskari P, Kangasdniemi P 1987 Response to occlusal treatment in headache patients previously treated by mock occlusal adjustment. Acta Odontologica Scandinavica 45:77–80

Pullinger A G, Seligman D A, Gornbein J A 1993 A multiple logistic regression analysis of the risk and relative odds of temporomandibular disorders as a function of common occlusal features. Journal of Dental Research 72:968–979

Tsukiyama Y, Baba K, Clark G T 2001 An evidence-based assessment of occlusal adjustment as a treatment for temporomandibular disorders. Journal of Prosthetic Dentistry 86:57–66

Further reading

Branam S R, Mourino A P 1998 Minimizing otitis media by manipulating the primary dental occlusion: case report. Journal of Clinical Pediatric Dentistry 22:203–206

Davies S J, Gray R M J, Smith P W 2001 Good occlusal practice in simple restorative dentistry. British Dental Journal 191:365–381

Gher M E 1998 Changing concepts. The effects of occlusion on periodontitis. Dental Clinics of North America 42:285–297

Greene C S, Laskin D M 2000 Temporomandibular disorders: moving from a dentally based to a medically based model. Journal of Dental Research 79:1736–1739

Hellsing G 1988 Occlusal adjustment and occlusal stability. Journal of Prosthetic Dentistry 59:696–702

Karjalainen M, Le Bell Y, Jamsa T, Karjalainen S 1997 Prevention of temporomandibular disorder-related signs and symptoms in orthodontically treated adolescents. A 3-year follow-up of a prospective randomized trial. Acta Odontologica Scandinavica 55:319–324

Kopp S, Wenneberg B 1981 Effects of occlusal treatment and intra-articular injections on temporomandibular joint pain and dysfunction. Acta Odontologica Scandinavica 39:87–96

Luther F 1998 Orthodontics and the temporomandibular joint: where are we now? Part 2. Functional occlusion, malocclusion, and TMD. Angle Orthodontist 68:305–316

Marklund S, Wänman A 2000 A century of controversy regarding the benefit or detriment of occlusal contacts on the mediotrusive side. Review. Journal of Oral Rehabilitation 27:553–562

Minagi S, Ohtsuki H, Sato T, Ishii A 1997 Effect of balancing-side occlusion on the ipsilateral TMJ dynamics under clenching. Journal of Oral Rehabilitation 24:57–62

Rosenberg P A, Babick P J, Schertzer L, Leung A 1998 The effect of occlusal reduction on pain after endodontic instrumentation. Journal of Endodontics 24:492–496

Tsolka P, Morris R W, Preiskel H W 1992 Occlusal adjustment therapy for craniomandibular disorders: a clinical assessment by a double-blind method. Journal of Prosthetic Dentistry 68:957–964

Vallon D, Ekberg E C, Nilner M, Kopp S 1995 Short-term effect of occlusal adjustment on craniomandibular disorders including headaches. Acta Odontologica Scandinavica 53:55–59

Index